Praise for *The FibroManual*

"*The FibroManual* is a real winner. Bringing together the best of conventional Western medicine and effective integrative approaches, it is hands down the most comprehensive book ever written on this subject. It will help thousands get better."

—CHRISTIANE NORTHRUP, MD, *New York Times* bestselling author of *Women's Bodies, Women's Wisdom*

"*The FibroManual* offers solid hope of living well with fibromyalgia. It includes valuable, insightful resources that reveal new integrative treatment options. People with fibromyalgia can feel confident in using Dr. Liptan's science-based treatment protocols. *The FibroManual* should be the first book to read for people who are newly diagnosed."

—JAN FAVERO CHAMBERS, president/founder, National Fibromyalgia & Chronic Pain Association

"*The FibroManual* includes all the little things that have made the biggest difference in my own fibromyalgia— treatments that took me years to find on my own as a patient. This book will be required reading for my students."

—TAMI STACKELHOUSE, founder, International Fibromyalgia Coaching Institute

"An inspiring story about how a physician overcame her own fibromyalgia, this book contains important lessons for both doctors and patients, as well as lots of practical advice and excellent references if you wish to dig deeper."
—RICHARD PODELL, MD, MPH, clinical professor, Department of Family Medicine and Community Health, Rutgers Robert Wood Johnson Medical School

"An easy-to-understand and well-referenced guide. Readers will find the answers they need to significantly improve their lives, and their care providers will find specific guidelines on therapies, medications, and supplements. I hope that they read this valuable book thoroughly, and that they keep it handy for frequent reference."
—DEVIN J. STARLANYL, co-author of *Fibromyalgia & Chronic Myofascial Pain Syndrome: A Survival Manual*

"Stop searching, the answers are all here! *The FibroManual* is a treasure trove of scientifically proven strategies to help both patients and providers understand and treat fibromyalgia. There is a lag between what scientists know and what your health care provider may know. Dr. Ginevra Liptan is here to help you bridge that gap with the easily understandable and accurate information in this book."
—KIM DUPREE JONES, PhD, FNP, FAAN, associate professor, School of Nursing, Oregon Health & Science University

"At last, here's a book with a practical and current map for managing all our fibromyalgia symptoms and an understanding that treatment should not follow a one-size-fits-all approach! I take this book to every appointment with my health care team."
—MELISSA TALWAR, director of patient advocacy and communications, National Fibromyalgia Association

The FibroManual

The FibroManual

A Complete Fibromyalgia Treatment Guide
for You *and* Your Doctor

GINEVRA LIPTAN, M.D.

BALLANTINE BOOKS
NEW YORK

No book can replace the diagnostic expertise and medical advice of a trusted physician. Please be certain to consult with your doctor before making any decisions that affect your health, particularly if you suffer from any medical condition or have any symptom that may require treatment.

As of the time of initial publication, the URLs displayed in this book link or refer to existing websites on the Internet. Penguin Random House LLC is not responsible for, and should not be deemed to endorse or recommend, any website other than its own or any content available on the Internet (including without limitation at any website, blog page, information page) that is not created by Penguin Random House.

A Ballantine Books Trade Paperback Original

Published in the United States by Ballantine Books,
an imprint of Random House, a division of
Penguin Random House LLC, New York.

BALLANTINE and the HOUSE colophon are
registered trademarks of Penguin Random House LLC.

Library of Congress Cataloging-in-Publication Data
Names: Liptan, Ginevra, author.
Title: The fibromanual : a complete fibromyalgia treatment guide for you and your doctor / Ginevra Liptan, M.D.
Description: New York : Ballantine Books, [2016] | "A Ballantine Books Trade Paperback Original."—Title page verso. | Includes bibliographical references and index.
Identifiers: LCCN 2016000491 (print) | LCCN 2016001478 (ebook) | ISBN 9781101967201 (paperback) | ISBN 9781101967218 (ebook)
Subjects: LCSH: Fibromyalgia—Treatment—Popular works. | Fibromyalgia—Handbooks, manuals, etc. | BISAC: HEALTH & FITNESS / Diseases / Musculoskeletal. | HEALTH & FITNESS / Healing. | HEALTH & FITNESS / Pain Management.
Classification: LCC RC927.3 .L57 2016 (print) | LCC RC927.3 (ebook) | DDC 616.7/42—dc23
LC record available at http://lccn.loc.gov/2016000491

Printed in the United States of America on acid-free paper

randomhousebooks.com

9 8 7 6 5 4 3 2 1

Book design by Diane Hobbing
Drawings by Bonnie Hofkin; flowcharts by Visible Logic, Inc.

For Dad

CONTENTS

INTRODUCTION

The F-Word

When describing fibromyalgia to someone without the condition, I ask them to recall the muscle soreness that follows a flu shot—then to imagine that ache throughout their whole body, along with profound fatigue and mental fog. I might show them the best visual depiction of this pain that I have seen: *The Broken Column,* a self-portrait by the Mexican painter and fibromyalgia sufferer Frida Kahlo, in which her body is pierced by nails (Martínez-Lavín 2000).

The ten million Americans currently struggling with these debilitating symptoms get very little help from their doctors. Research has lagged far behind other diseases, bogged down by controversy and a century of arguments about whether it is a "real" illness. The fact that it primarily affects women has contributed to its categorization as a second-class or "wastebasket" diagnosis. The stigma attached to fibromyalgia—both having it and treating it—is why I half-seriously refer to it as the F-word of medicine.

Although more than six thousand studies have now illuminated the processes in the body that cause fibromyalgia and provided effective options for treatment, many physicians still don't understand it well enough to assist their patients (Hadker 2011; Perrot 2012). This leaves sufferers desperately trying to figure it out on their own, which is exactly what I experienced after developing fibromyalgia in my second year of medical school. This book provides all the information I needed back then, including research-supported medical guidance to bring to your doctor's attention and specific advice on practical things you can do for yourself.

A Doctor with an Invisible Illness

At age twenty-six, I suddenly went from being a healthy and active (if overworked and poorly rested) medical student to barely functional, exhausted, and in pain all the time. I attributed it to the stress and long hours of school, so I tried to eat better and sleep more. But I just kept getting worse. I made appointments with some of the top specialists in Boston; none of them could figure out what was wrong. I saw alternative medical practitioners, including acupuncturists and naturopaths and a well-regarded holistic MD, but still no answers.

I was ultimately diagnosed by a chiropractor. Finally having a name for what I was going through was a relief, but then things went from bad to worse. One day during teaching rounds, my senior physician authoritatively announced, "Fibromyalgia does not exist." I realized that many doctors, even my closest friends, dismissed sufferers as hypochondriacs. I told no one about my illness and was left to fend for myself with Dr. Google and self-help books.

Medicine had failed me. I had to figure it out for myself, which remains an all too common situation for people with the condition. I was fortunate, however, to have the training to interpret research studies and find and access cutting-edge treatments. Using myself as a guinea pig, I eventually found some very effective regimens, which I have now used to treat thousands of patients. I discovered that gaining real improvement in symptoms requires an integrative approach that includes *both* Western and alternative treatments.

My med school and residency training was purely Western medicine, but since then I have studied integrative therapies through the Institute for Functional Medicine. I have treated fibromyalgia as a primary care provider, a pain specialist, and in the rheumatology clinic at Oregon Health and Science University. But it is my personal experience that gives me the unique perspective of a physician studying this illness from the inside.

Fibromyalgia Is Real and Can Be Treated

In 2002 a groundbreaking study showed abnormalities in how the brain processes pain in fibromyalgia (Gracely 2002). This research finally provided the objective data to prove fibromyalgia was "real," and gave a target for drug development. A decade of intensive research resulted in three FDA-approved drugs that dull the pain signals in the brain. But those medications don't treat the often more debilitating symptoms of fatigue and fuzzy thinking called "fibrofog."

In fact, pain-processing problems are only the tip of the iceberg. A much bigger factor is a stress (or danger) response that has gone haywire and is constantly on red alert, leading to a chain reaction that results in fatigue, brain fog, and muscle pain. The only way to get lasting improvement in all of these symptoms is to systematically address the negative effects on the body of a chronic hyperactive stress response. My treatment approach does this in four manageable steps, which I call the four R's:

- First, **Rest:** give the body a break from the constant pummeling by a hyperactive stress response by purposefully enlisting a relaxation response and by restoring deep sleep.

- Once the foundation of **Rest** is in place, we add **Repair,** both structural and nutritional. The stress response weakens the body's ability to break down and absorb nutrients, so we fix digestion. Muscle pain is eased with gentle movement and myofascial release, a specialized manual therapy that targets painful connective tissue.
- The next step is to **Rebalance** the problems with energy production, hormones, and inflammation caused by a chronic stress response.
- Finally, **Reduce** any remaining pain, fatigue, or fibrofog by treating specific symptoms with targeted medications and therapies.

Helping Your Doctor to Help You

At this point you may be wondering, "If there are all these effective treatments out there, why doesn't my doctor know about them?" Certainly, the F-word stigma contributes to this gap in knowledge, but fibromyalgia is also an orphan disease that is not claimed by a specialty and instead awkwardly straddles the fields of rheumatology, neurology, and sleep and pain medicine. The majority of care falls to overwhelmed primary care doctors who don't have time to go searching for new treatment ideas among the sea of medical publications. Add in the common delays between research findings and adoption into clinical practice, and you can see why the average health care provider has little to offer.

The typical research-to-practice gap is exacerbated by the lack of space for fibromyalgia in the big medical journals. Since 1987, only one fibromyalgia study has been published in the *New England Journal of Medicine,* the most widely read medical publication in the world. Some helpful treatments are neglected because they involve unusual uses of medications, like the dementia drug that dramatically reduces fibromyalgia pain and brain fog. Others are ignored because they come from the world of alternative medicine. Doctors simply don't read massage therapy journals, like the one that published a large European study showing that myofascial release therapy provided long-lasting relief from fibromyalgia pain.

Since the average busy primary care provider does not have time to actively search out studies on new treatments, research has to be brought to their attention in some other way—namely by their patients. As a practicing physician myself, I know how to get your doctor's attention. The appendix contains a research-supported guide to share with your health care provider.

Some of my recommendations are "clinical pearls" that aren't found in any textbook, but rather are gained only through experience during medical training. Others are hidden gems, studies that show good results of a treatment or medication but may get lost in the sea of information and never make it onto a doctor's radar. Bringing these to your doctor's attention allows her to provide you with expert-level fibromyalgia care.

Is There a Cure?

There is no cure for fibromyalgia, yet. But we don't have cures for many chronic illnesses, like diabetes and high blood pressure—what we *do* have are effective treatments that manage those diseases well enough that they are minimally detrimental to one's health. And powerful treatments for fibromyalgia are out there as well.

When people ask me if I have recovered from fibromyalgia, I say, "Yes." I have found ways to feel much better and minimize its impact on my life. Ultimately, I do still have fibromyalgia, and there is no magic bullet that completely eliminates all symptoms. It requires work, and I have learned that consistency in my self-care routine is essential. With the tools in these pages, you'll learn how to help yourself—and enable your doctor to help you—to dramatically reduce your symptoms too.

The FibroManual

_____

CHAPTER 1

Figuring Out Fibromyalgia for Myself

At the end of my first year of medical school, I was doing crunches at the gym when I felt a muscle in the front of my neck rip, causing intense pain. I had injured muscles before, and I figured it would heal quickly. But as days turned to weeks, it didn't. My neck burned constantly and felt like it could no longer hold up the weight of my head. The only relief I got was when I wrapped a heating pad around it. A chiropractor found mild abnormalities in my cervical spine and made some adjustments. I started getting regular chiropractic treatments, because they were all I could think to do, and they helped a little.

That summer, I was achy and tired all the time. I took a part-time babysitting job, and working for just a few hours left me exhausted for days. I woke up in the morning with a sore neck and back, which hurt all day. I frequently felt stiff, weak, and lightheaded. It was as if all the energy of my body and mind had been sucked out. I went to see my primary care doctor, who prescribed a muscle relaxant, which did not help. The pain progressed to my upper back—an ache between my shoulder blades that would not go away. My spine hurt, my skin hurt, everything hurt. I was sleeping poorly, tossing and turning, and I woke every morning feeling more tired than before I went to bed. I felt too weak to even lift my arms to wash my hair in the shower.

One day my hips started aching so much that I couldn't do anything but lie in bed and cry. I was sure there was something really wrong with me, so I went again to my doctor. She drew blood and sent me to a rheumatologist. The rheumatologist ordered X-rays of my neck and hips and assured me they were completely normal.

"So why do I hurt all the time?" I asked.

"I don't know, but you don't have arthritis," he responded.

I returned to my doctor to find that my labs were all normal. My doctors had no answers for me and nothing to offer.

A Diagnosis

I started my second year of medical school as a total wreck. And then a bit of grace fell my way. My chiropractor sold her practice. I tearfully told my entire story to the chiropractor who took it over, and he suggested that I might have fibromyalgia—the first time anyone had even mentioned it to me. He checked my tender points, and registered "exquisite" tenderness in at least twelve of them, confirming the diagnosis. He recommended that I pick up what he called "the bible of fibromyalgia," *Fibromyalgia and Chronic Myofascial Pain Syndrome: A Survival Manual,* by Devin Starlanyl and Mary Ellen Copeland. I spent weeks reading and rereading it, trying to convince myself that I did not have the condition, but unable to avoid the fact that it described me perfectly. "Chronic" was such an awful word. And fibromyalgia had such a stigma among doctors—even among my fellow medical students—that I couldn't quite believe I had it.

I began doing research in my medical textbooks, on the Internet, and in bookstores. I quickly became discouraged. Western medicine had little to offer beyond antidepressants and exercise. I was already on antidepressants, and exercise made me feel worse. So I ventured into the confusing world of alternative medicine, perusing countless theories and treatments online, many of which conflicted directly with what I was learning in school. I was overwhelmed by the different ideas I encountered about the causes of fibromyalgia and how to treat it.

Was it yeast overgrowth? Low thyroid hormone production? Did I need to cleanse my body of toxins? Do a raw-juice fast? Use guaifenesin to reduce calcium phosphate deposits in the muscles? Was I deficient in some vitamin that I needed in megadoses? Did I need a macrobiotic diet? Raw foods? Alkaline foods?

Compounding my frustration was the fact that I was so fatigued I didn't have the energy to contemplate major lifestyle or dietary changes. Acupuncture didn't help, and massage made me feel more achy and tired. The latter half of my second year of medical school was basically a very expensive correspondence course. I rarely felt well enough to make it to class, and survived by getting lecture notes from friends, studying at home, and showing up only for the occasional required seminar and exams.

I finally accepted that I had fibromyalgia. I felt hopeless and helpless. I told myself that it wasn't fatal—it wasn't *cancer*—but it still felt like a death sentence. It became clear that there was no way I could make it through the rigors of the third year of medical school, with its eighty-hour workweeks and high levels of physical and emotional stress. I took a leave of absence.

Stumbling into Help

During my yearlong leave I read every book I could get my hands on about fibromyalgia and tried every treatment I could. I knew exercise was supposed to help, so I kept trying new regimens, only to stop after injuring myself. After diligently following the guaifenesin protocol described in *What Your Doctor*

May Not Tell You About Fibromyalgia: The Revolutionary Treatment That Can Reverse the Disease, by R. Paul St. Amand and Claudi Craig Marek, I was devastated when I got no benefit from it. I took thousands of dollars' worth of useless supplements. I tried IV therapies with a naturopath, and saw a top holistic MD in Boston. I did colonic hydrotherapy and fasted and did detoxifying diets. I tried every type of massage I could find, but each session seemed to make my pain worse. I journaled and saw a therapist and tried to meditate. None of it helped, and midway through the year I was feeling hopeless and preparing to drop out of school completely.

Then I read Claire Musickant's *Fibromyalgia: My Journey to Wellness.* Musickant describes her dramatic reduction in symptoms after testing for food sensitivities and eliminating the offenders. I knew it was something I needed to do; it felt right. I had a rare rush of hope and excitement as I called the lab to find a practitioner in my area, a naturopath. She told me the test was expensive. I hesitated and asked her if she had found that it helped people with fibromyalgia. "Oh, yes," she said, "and it helped me. I had fibromyalgia and am now ninety percent better." She *had* fibromyalgia—*past tense.* These were possibly the most beautiful words I had ever heard. She was the first person I had talked to who had even suggested that fibromyalgia was something one could recover from.

I did the blood test and started to avoid the recommended foods and chemicals. After about two weeks, I realized that the all-over body ache I had grown so accustomed to was gone. Now it only hurt when someone actually pressed on my muscles. It didn't feel as if I constantly had the flu. I had the energy to grocery shop, to cook, to exercise. I was thrilled. But my sleep was still light and restless and I woke up exhausted every morning. My neck and arm pain flared up easily with exertion or repeated motion.

A massage therapist recommended I try a manual therapy

technique, the John F. Barnes' Myofascial Release Approach, which involves slow, prolonged stretching that releases restrictions in the fascia, the connective tissue around the muscle (see chapter 12 for further details). After several sessions I experienced dramatic pain reduction in my arms and neck. With ongoing myofascial release therapy, I felt well enough to return to medical school, but I remained fatigued all the time. Things really fell apart during a month of night shifts in the hospital. I couldn't sleep during the day and developed severe insomnia. I dragged myself once again to my primary doctor, who prescribed a sleep medication.

Suddenly everything shifted. I was getting deeper sleep and feeling more rested when I woke up. The combination of improving sleep quality with medication, avoiding inflammation-producing foods, and myofascial release treatments got me through the grueling remainder of medical school and residency training. And it forms the core of my treatment approach to this day. Over the years I fine-tuned my technique, learning other ways to improve deep sleep, treat the fascia, and warm up so that exercise helps and doesn't hurt.

As I continued my medical training, I was able to better assess the thousands of studies and articles written about fibromyalgia. I began to put together why certain treatments had helped me so much, while others did nothing at all. Based on my own relief with myofascial release I was convinced that the fascia was the source of fibromyalgia pain, and my research has focused on it ever since. At Oregon Health and Science University I conducted a study that found myofascial release therapy was more helpful than standard massage for fibromyalgia symptoms (Liptan 2013). I've also published articles on exercise and self-management strategies (Jones 2012; Liptan 2010; Jones 2009). In 2011 I founded the first private practice in the United States dedicated exclusively to fibromyalgia, the Frida Center for Fibromyalgia, in Lake Oswego, Oregon.

For years after my diagnosis I felt bitter toward all the doctors who had not been able to help me. It was so frustrating that again and again I had to find my own way, wasting money on ineffective treatments because I had no guidance. My resentment faded, though, as I continued my medical training and practice and realized that physicians in this country are working within an untenable system. Our current medical framework is just not set up well to deal with chronic and complex illnesses like fibromyalgia. And while most doctors do really try to help their fibromyalgia patients, they simply lack the expertise or tools to do it.

I told no one about my diagnosis, even my closest friends. I only revealed it during my final presentation to colleagues and teachers on the last day of my residency. I felt as if I was "coming out" and revealing a whole secret life. I wanted to show my fellow doctors it is a real disease that can happen to anyone. Since then, I have focused a large part of my career on educating other health care professionals about this invisible illness. I am done feeling ashamed. My hypervigilant nervous system keeps me attuned to subtle changes in other people's emotional states and in my environment. It has helped me to become a better doctor. And my intimate experiences with pain and suffering have made me a better human being.

CHAPTER 2

What Fibromyalgia Is—and Isn't

Fibromyalgia is extremely common, affecting at least 3 percent of the population in the United States (Lawrence 1998; White 1999). The typical sufferer is an otherwise healthy young woman in her twenties or thirties. It doesn't discriminate by socioeconomic class: my patients include fast-food workers, lawyers, custodians, school district superintendents, zookeepers, and teachers. While it predominantly affects women, many more men, especially combat veterans, have been diagnosed in recent years.

Most patients first seek medical guidance for persistent pain or fatigue, but they may also experience irritable bowel and bladder symptoms, low blood pressure, dizziness on standing, poor balance, frequent headaches, numbness or tingling in hands or feet, and sensitivity to loud noises. All of these symptoms can be tied in one way or another to dysfunction in the stress response.

Given the prevalence of fibromyalgia and how much research has now been done, it seems like it should be easy for health care providers to diagnose, doesn't it? Unfortunately, that's not the case, because there are no accepted imaging or blood tests that can confirm a diagnosis. Complicating matters, its symptoms are not unique; similar problems can be caused by anemia, hypothyroidism, and chronic fatigue syndrome. If you see your doctor for fatigue or muscle pain, the workup usually starts with lab tests for thyroid function, red blood cell count, and inflammation in the blood as she tries to rule out other potential causes. Standard laboratory tests come back *normal* in fibromyalgia, so it is considered a diagnosis of exclusion, given only after no other sources of muscle pain and fatigue have been found.

Fibromyalgia Is a Clinical Diagnosis

The lack of lab abnormalities associated with fibromyalgia, and the fact that sufferers don't "look sick," have contributed to the controversy surrounding this illness. Technically, fibromyalgia is not even considered a disease; it is still referred to in the medical literature as a *syndrome:* a collection of signs, symptoms, and medical problems that tend to occur together but are not related to a specific, identifiable cause. A *disease,* meanwhile, has a specific cause or causes and recognizable signs and symptoms. As you will learn, I do feel that there is a specific cause for fibromyalgia and thus refer to it as a disease or illness throughout this book.

To ease the difficulty of diagnosing fibromyalgia, in 1990 a group of rheumatologists created a set of diagnostic criteria for doctors and researchers (Wolfe 1990). Patients with fibromyalgia have "widespread pain in multiple connective tissue areas" (Mease 2011), and through trial and error these rheumatologists found that most patients were very tender in eighteen specific points in the muscles: on both sides of the body, just under the knees and elbows, in the lower back and gluteal region, and in the neck and over the second ribs, near the breastbone. To be diagnosed with fibromyalgia, you need a history of diffuse musculoskeletal pain and tenderness on palpation (applied pressure) in eleven of those eighteen points.

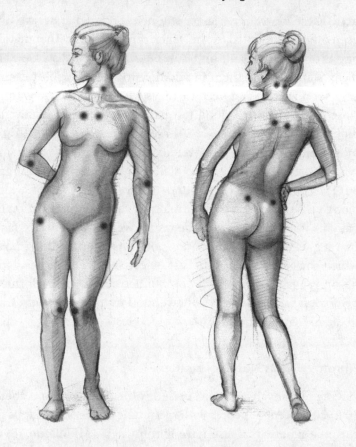

The eighteen tender points used to diagnose fibromyalgia.

Over the years there has been increased recognition that fatigue, poor sleep, and cognitive dysfunction ("fibrofog") almost always accompany the muscle pain in fibromyalgia. So in 2010 a different team of rheumatologists developed another diagnostic tool (Wolfe 2011) that no longer requires a tender point exam. Instead, a patient must describe widespread pain in specific areas of the body and moderate to severe symptoms of fatigue, waking unrefreshed from sleep, and cognitive dysfunction. These newer criteria are still being refined and have not been officially adopted by the American College of Rheumatology as of the writing of this book, but many specialists have already started using them in addition to a tender point exam. And soon we may not need them, as we are—happily—getting close to a diagnostic blood test based on the work of several different research groups. In 2014 researchers at Virginia Commonwealth University discovered a specific pattern of inflammatory chemicals in the blood of fibromyalgia subjects (Sturgill 2014). Other researchers found that certain types of white blood cells do not respond normally to chemical stimulation in patients with fibromyalgia. The results were so striking, in fact, that it was developed into a test for consumers, called FM/a, which they are calling "the first objective diagnostic test" for fibromyalgia (Behm 2012). More studies need to be performed before it is widely adopted, but we soon may finally have a way to diagnose fibromyalgia from a blood test.

Fibromyalgia Is Not Exclusionary

Having fibromyalgia doesn't exclude other ailments, and about 10 to 20 percent of people with rheumatic diseases like lupus or rheumatoid arthritis also have fibromyalgia (Middleton 1994; Haliloglu 2014). Lupus and rheumatoid arthritis are autoimmune diseases in which the immune system attacks the body. In rheumatoid arthritis this causes severe joint inflammation, especially in the hands and feet. In lupus it results in facial rash and diffuse joint pain, and can also cause blood clots and kidney problems. Many people with fibromyalgia wonder if they may also have an autoimmune illness, and blood tests to rule them out are part of the standard workup. Keep in mind that it is possible to have both fibromyalgia and lupus, or both fibromyalgia and rheumatoid arthritis.

Fibromyalgia can also be triggered by other illnesses, such

as Lyme disease or chronic fatigue syndrome (Dinerman 1992). In fact, I estimate that about 15 percent of my fibromyalgia patients also have chronic fatigue syndrome. These overlapping illnesses can make it hard for your health care provider to make an accurate diagnosis since many Western or conventionally trained providers are not knowledgeable about chronic fatigue syndrome or Lyme disease. I will delineate the differences between fibromyalgia and chronic Lyme disease and chronic fatigue syndrome for your understanding. If you suspect you may have either, I recommend consulting a naturopath or a provider who specializes in their treatment.

Fibromyalgia Versus Chronic Fatigue Syndrome

Doctors and patients alike are confused by the similarities between chronic fatigue syndrome (CFS) and fibromyalgia (FM). Both are poorly understood conditions that are characterized by fatigue and primarily affect women. Complicating matters further, the two terms are often used interchangeably or lumped together and treated as if they were the same disease, under the banner of "FM/CFS." Many of my patients think they must have chronic fatigue syndrome because they feel fatigued all the time, and this is a common misperception. But there are actually very specific criteria for CFS—it has unique symptoms, different triggers (for example, the fatigue stems from a dysfunctional immune system), and responds to different treatments. Most CFS patients describe a sudden onset of symptoms, often after a flulike illness, suggesting that it may be triggered by an infection. For the past thirty years, researchers have theorized that it is caused by a viral infection because of certain telltale changes seen in the blood and immune cells of CFS patients. However, no one has been able to identify a specific instigating virus, so it is now thought that a few different types of viral infections may trigger the immune system to go haywire.

It is this overactive immune response, not a viral infection, that leads to fatigue, low-grade fevers, sore throat, and swollen lymph nodes. Fibromyalgia, on the other hand, usually has a gradual onset, and is not associated with fevers, sore throats, or lymph node swelling.

For patients with both fibromyalgia and chronic fatigue syndrome, I find that they still need my complete four R's regimen, but also benefit from addressing any immune system problems directly. See chapter 23 for details on this treatment.

Fibromyalgia Versus Chronic Lyme Disease

Chronic Lyme disease refers to long-lasting symptoms stemming from infection with the spiral-shaped bacteria called *Borrelia burgdorferi* that causes acute Lyme disease. Acute Lyme disease is transmitted to people via deer tick bites and causes fever, headache, and a characteristic skin rash that looks like a bull's-eye. If caught early, it can be treated with a round of antibiotics. But if left untreated (or if the infected person is unaware they have it), it can spread throughout the body and have long-lasting effects. Around three hundred thousand people in the United States are diagnosed with acute Lyme disease annually, mostly in New England and the upper Midwest (CDC 2013).

Ten to fifteen percent of people who are treated for Lyme disease develop persistent or recurrent symptoms of fatigue, migratory joint and muscle pain, headaches, and neurologic abnormalities like confusion and tingling, numbness, and burning or stabbing sensations. This is known as post-treatment Lyme disease syndrome (PTLDS). These patients' blood tests are often negative for Lyme, so most doctors do not continue to administer antibiotics, but instead will just treat their symptoms. However, many alternative practitioners and Lyme specialists believe that the bacteria may still be present even if it isn't showing up on standard blood tests, and they'll treat it with long-term antibiotics, sometimes for several years. Best practices for Lyme remain a hotly argued and very controversial area of medicine.

The crux of the debate is that the available blood tests for Lyme disease are not very accurate. Generally, the best way to test for infection is to take a blood or fluid sample and see what bacteria grow from it. But the Lyme bacteria is very hard to grow in the lab, so instead we look for antibodies to the bacteria using a two-tier method of blood tests: the first detects the presence of antibodies, and if they are found, the sample is analyzed further to get a breakdown of how many and what types are present. A patient must test positive on both tiers to be officially diagnosed with Lyme.

The International Lyme and Associated Diseases Society estimates that these antibody tests are wrong about 40 percent of the time. Instead of relying exclusively on those results, the society emphasizes the importance of a doctor's clinical judgment. If you are concerned that you may have chronic Lyme disease, I highly recommend you find a knowledgeable practitioner, a "Lyme-literate doctor." In my region this is usually a naturopath, but it will vary from state to state, especially as more MDs learn about diagnosis and treatment on the East Coast in particular.

With symptoms that are so similar to fibromyalgia, you can see why chronic Lyme disease might easily be misdiagnosed, especially if the patient doesn't recall a tick bite. And of course, Lyme can trigger the onset of fibromyalgia, so someone can have both diseases at once. One clinic reported that of 287 patients seen with chronic Lyme disease, 22 (8 percent) also had fibromyalgia (Dinerman 1992). As with CFS, if you have chronic Lyme disease, you will benefit from my four R's treatment program but will also likely require additional therapies specific to the illness.

If you think you might have fibromyalgia, please see your

health care provider to confirm the diagnosis and make sure she fully rules out any of the mimics like anemia and hypothyroidism, and determines whether you may have an overlapping illness like chronic fatigue syndrome, chronic Lyme disease, lupus, or rheumatoid arthritis. To be fully evaluated, consider seeing a specialist such as a rheumatologist or infectious disease doctor.

Chapter Resources

- IGeneX (www.igenex.com) is a laboratory specializing in testing for Lyme and tick-borne illness.
- The International Lyme and Associated Diseases Society website (www.ilads.org) has good information about diagnosis and treatment.
- Visit www.lymediseaseassociation.org to find Lyme-literate providers in your area.

Good Books on Lyme Disease

Why Can't I Get Better? Solving the Mystery of Lyme and Chronic Disease by Richard Horowitz, MD.

Cure Unknown: Inside the Lyme Epidemic by Pamela Weintraub, revised edition.

CHAPTER 3

The Chain Reaction That Causes Fibromyalgia

Anyone who has seen a TV advertisement for a fibromyalgia drug has heard that the ailment is caused by "overactivity of pain-sensing nerves." And it's true that when the brain and spinal cord increase the volume on pain signals as in fibromyalgia, the result is pain hypersensitivity—the target of the three FDA-approved medications for this illness. But that's just the tip of the iceberg. The crucial thing to remember with fibromyalgia is that the nervous system is stuck in the stress response (Martínez-Lavín 2012, 1998). In fact, *all* symptoms of fibromyalgia, including excessive pain, are the result of a complex chain reaction set off by a hyperactive stress response.

The stress response is an automatic brain reflex that is commonly referred to as the "fight or flight" instinct. It has little to do with feeling stressed out. Rather, it refers to the body's automatic response to danger, triggered by a primal brain area whose only focus is on survival. When a potential threat is detected—a loud banging on your front door, a stranger moving quickly toward you on the street—the brain prepares the body by pumping adrenaline and tightening muscles, readying your whole system for action. This is the body's normal response to danger—great for a short-term response, and activated only when there is an imminent threat. In fibromyalgia, however, the stress response never stops, like a smoke alarm that goes off incessantly even though there's no fire.

When chronically activated, it wreaks havoc on the body, preventing deep sleep; keeping muscles tense, leading to pain and tenderness; impairing digestion and energy production; and throwing hormones out of balance. It also ultimately causes the pain-sensing nerves to increase the volume of their signals. (For more information about the chain reaction set off by the hyperactive stress response, check out chapter 7.)

To treat fibromyalgia we have to stop this chain reaction at the source by blocking the hyperactive stress response. In order to understand how, let's dive deeper into its wide-ranging effects.

The "Autopilot" Nervous System

The nervous system consists of the brain, the spinal cord, and the nerves. A network of nerves known as the autonomic nervous system controls the housekeeping functions of the body such as blood pressure, heart rate, breathing, digestion, and urination. Its job is to be the "autopilot" that controls the most basic survival functions of the body. The autonomic nervous system is controlled by areas deep in the brain stem, in the "animal" or primal part of our brain that is not under our conscious control. It's the region that can keep someone with a massive head injury alive and breathing in a vegetative state.

Branching out from the control center in the brain stem are two bundles of nerves that each extend to the entire body but with opposing functions. One branch is the sympathetic nerves that prepare the body for action by tensing the muscles, dilating the pupils, and increasing the heart rate in the face of a threat. The other is the parasympathetic nerves that prepare the body for rest, by relaxing muscles, slowing the heart rate, and dilating blood vessels. The brain stem is constantly shifting the balance between these contrary responses, which is how it keeps all the autopilot systems running smoothly. When you drive a car, you modulate the gas pedal and brake to control your speed. Likewise, when the brain stem activates the sympathetic branch it is pressing on the gas pedal, and when it activates the parasympathetic branch it is stepping on the brake.

Opposing Actions of the Two Branches of the Autonomic Nervous System

Sympathetic (Fight-or-Flight) Nervous System	Parasympathetic (Rest-and-Digest) Nervous System
• Tunes all body systems for a stress response. • Increases attention/hypervigilance. • Tenses muscles. • Dilates pupils. • Increases heart rate and force. • Diverts blood flow away from gastrointestinal system. • Reduces gastric secretions. • Slows gastric motility. • Constricts blood vessels. • Increases fuel metabolism to give burst of strength and energy.	• Tunes all body systems for a relaxation response. • Calms brain/decreases vigilance. • Relaxes muscles. • Constricts pupils. • Decreases heart rate and force. • Increases blood flow to gastrointestinal system. • Increases gastric secretions. • Quickens gastric motility. • Relaxes blood vessels. • Slows fuel metabolism to resting state.

The baseline mode of the autopilot system is rest-and-digest, but it shifts into the fight-or-flight mode as needed. For example, standing up would cause a big drop in your blood pressure if the brain stem didn't briefly activate the sympathetic nervous system to constrict blood vessels in your legs. However, the most important and complex role of the autopilot nervous system is to regulate the body's response to danger through the stress response.

Understanding the Stress Response

The hypothalamus, an area deep in the brain, acts as the command center for the stress response. If it senses danger, it sends a message to the adrenal glands telling them to pump out cortisol and adrenaline, the stress hormones that help marshal the body's resources to fight off or run away from a threat. Next, it sends an alarm signal down the brain stem to hit the gas pedal hard. This activates the sympathetic nerves throughout the body, causing blood vessels to clamp down and divert blood flow away from nonessential activities like digestion and urination. Sympathetic nerves tense the muscles to prepare to fight or run. They make the heart pound and the skin sweat. They increase attention in the brain, causing a state of hypervigilance. Together, the hypothalamus, brain stem, and sympathetic nerves are called the sympathetic, or "fight or flight," nervous system.

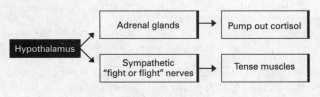

The stress response.

Because the ability to sense and respond to danger is essential for survival, the stress response involves almost every system in coordination. The brain stem and sympathetic nerves communicate with the immune system and with the network of pain-sensing nerves throughout the body. Once a threat has passed, the brain stem calls off the fight-or-flight response, pressing the brake and activating the parasympathetic, or "rest and digest," nerves to switch the body's systems back into nondanger or rest mode: shifting blood flow back to digestion and urination, relaxing the muscles, slowing the heart rate, and calming the brain.

Triggers of the Abnormal Stress Response in Fibromyalgia

We don't know for certain exactly how or why the hypothalamus gets stuck sounding the alarm and continually activating the stress response in fibromyalgia. There seems to be a genetic component; fibromyalgia tends to run in families just like diabetes and many other chronic illnesses (Arnold 2004). Fibromyalgia patients are more likely to carry genes for a dysfunctional enzyme that normally breaks down the chemical messengers of the fight-or-flight nervous system. (Martinez-Jauand 2013; Barbosa 2012; Cohen 2009; Desmeules 2014). They are also more likely to have genes that code for abnormal receptors in fight-or-flight nerves (Vargas-Alarcón 2009; Maekawa 2003; Xiao 2011).

There are also psychological risk factors for fibromyalgia, including childhood trauma or abuse (Greenfield 1992; White 1999). More than half of women with fibromyalgia report childhood sexual abuse, and 90 percent have experienced a sexual or physical assault in their lifetime (Walker 1997). There is an overlap with another disease closely linked to trauma, post-traumatic stress disorder (PTSD). Almost half of male patients with combat-related PTSD meet the diagnostic criteria for fibromyalgia (Amital 2006).

My own story follows a similar path to that of many of my patients; after suffering a sexual assault in adolescence, I was well positioned, from a clinical standpoint, to develop fibromyalgia.

The most widely accepted theory is that in genetically or psychologically predisposed people, a trauma in adulthood triggers a prolonged activation of the stress response system. In fact, a "physical trauma in the preceding six months is significantly associated with the onset of fibromyalgia" (Al-Allaf 2002). For me that trigger seems to have been the neck injury I sustained while weight lifting. Other potential triggers may include a major infection or illness, or prolonged pressure on the spinal cord in the neck. While most people with fibromyalgia can identify a provoking event such as an injury, car accident, or emotional trauma, not everyone does (Hryciw 2010; Holman 2008; Dinerman 1992; Buskila 1997).

Effects of Chronic Stress Response Activation on the Body

The stress response is designed to provide a temporary burst of activity to give us enough energy and time to either fight an attacker or run away. But when it is chronically activated, it sets off a chain reaction resulting in fatigue and muscle pain and, most damaging, constant activity of the fight-or-flight nerves. Brief fight-or-flight activation results in hypervigilance, making us more aware of our surroundings, and readies our muscles for action. Long-term activation causes poor sleep as the brain remains perpetually alert, and results in muscle tension and pain. It slows down digestion so over time the gastrointestinal system begins to function poorly. Finally, it can temporarily block pain signals, but chronic activation leads to *increased* pain intensity (Donello 2011).

The stress response is so overactive in fibromyalgia that it is less able to respond to actual threats; if the gas pedal is already pressed all the way to the floor, you can't pump it any harder to increase your speed. For example, an impaired ability to respond to stressors like infection is quite common (Elenkov 2000). Even bodily functions as simple as standing up can be dysfunctional. Normally, going from a seated to a standing position triggers the fight-or-flight nervous system to constrict the blood vessels in the legs to prevent a drop in blood pressure. In fibromyalgia, however, these nerves are already on overdrive, so they can't send the signal to the blood vessels to constrict, resulting in the common symptom of low blood pressure and dizziness upon standing (Bou-Holaigah 1997).

If we could find a way to reset the hypothalamus so that it was not constantly activating the stress response, we would have the cure for fibromyalgia. We haven't discovered that yet, so the key to treatment is to lessen the problems it causes. In the next chapter you will learn the most effective ways to block each step of the chain reaction and reduce your symptoms.

CHAPTER 4

Blocking the Fibromyalgia Chain Reaction

The chain reaction of fibromyalgia begins with excessive activation of the stress response, which prevents deep sleep, impairs growth hormone release, and leads to tense and inflamed muscles. That inflammation is primarily in the surrounding connective tissue, or fascia, an area rich with pain-sensing nerves. Hyperactive fight-or-flight nerve signals combine with inflammation to agitate these pain-sensing nerves and stimulate louder pain signals. Those constant signals overwhelm the spinal cord and brain and induce a state of hyperreactivity to pain.

We don't yet have a way to permanently fix the chronic hyperactivity of the stress response, but by frequently shifting our body back into the rest-and-digest mode we can limit its negative effects. Next, we must override the stress response at night to allow the brain and body to fall into deep sleep. These vital steps form the foundation of fibromyalgia treatment and can lead to significant improvement in all the downstream complications caused by a stress response gone haywire. This chapter provides an overview so you can see how everything fits together. You will learn about each of these treatments in detail in the next section of the book.

Treatment starts with blocking the hyperactive stress response by activating its opposite: the relaxation response. Deep

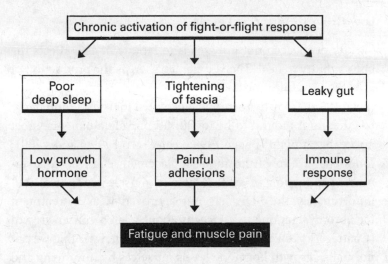

The chain reaction of fibromyalgia.

breathing and gentle stretching are two of your most powerful tools, but you will learn about many other easy ways to mobilize the beneficial rest-and-digest nerves.

Sleeping with One Eye Open

A brain sending danger signals does not allow itself to truly rest. Sleep, especially deep sleep, is a vulnerable time that is not compatible with fighting or fleeing! So fibromyalgia sleep is light and restless. One of my patients described it perfectly as "sleeping with one eye open." Sleep studies show that fibromyalgia subjects show abnormal "awake-type" brain waves all night long, with reduced and interrupted deep sleep and frequent "mini-awakenings" (Branco 1994; Kooh 2003). This deep-sleep deprivation leads to pain, fatigue, and poor brain function (Lerma 2011; Moldofsky 2008; Harding 1998). Treatment focused on increasing deep sleep is the key to improving all these symptoms.

Low Growth Hormone Levels

Lack of deep sleep not only leads to fatigue, it also affects the body's ability to heal. The key element here is the production of growth hormone, most of which occurs during deep sleep (Felig 1995). Growth hormone is essential for muscle and nerve health, and it's found to be low in fibromyalgia patients, most noticeably at night (Bagge 1998; Leal-Cerro 1999; Landis 2001; Jones 2007). Growth hormone replacement can lead to a significant reduction in symptoms and muscle tenderness, but unfortunately the FDA has not approved it as a treatment for fibromyalgia due to concerns about related cancer growth (Cuatrecasas 2007; Bennett 1998). The good news is that we can normalize growth hormone levels ourselves by improving and deepening our sleep.

Hormone Dysfunction

It is not just growth hormone that is altered in fibromyalgia. The secretion of cortisol, the stress hormone, is also affected (Mahdi 2011). The hyperactive stress response pushes the adrenal glands to their maximum output, which over time leads to adrenal glands that are not functioning well. Adrenal gland dysfunction causes fatigue, low blood pressure, and increased thirst. Specific treatments to support the adrenal glands are very effective in reducing these symptoms. The stress response also interferes with activation and absorption of thyroid hormones (Riedel 1998). Patients with hypothyroidism in addition to fibromyalgia often need a distinct regimen to get around this problem.

Muscle Tension

As part of the stress response, the brain sends signals to tighten the muscles and their surrounding connective tissues to increase their strength (Klingler 2014; Schleip 2005). In fibromyalgia there is no relief from this muscle tension (Bazzichi 2009; Anders 2001). Research shows that a pressure gauge needle inserted into fibromyalgia muscles shows increased pressure compared to healthy controls (Kokebie 2008). When the muscles and their surrounding connective tissue, called the fascia, are chronically tightened, as in fibromyalgia, they become inflamed and painful (Spaeth 2005; Rüster 2005). Manual therapies that reduce that tightness and painful inflammation are critical to recovery.

Muscle Energy Imbalance

Chronic fight-or-flight nerve activation depletes muscles of energy (Elenkov 2000; Gerdle 2013). Fight-or-flight nerves signal them to quickly burn through all their fuel in order to run away. But like a car with bad gas mileage, this is a very inefficient way to use fuel. This is why people with fibromyalgia have a reduced tolerance for exercise and their muscles get fatigued easily (Bachasson 2013; Park 1998; Shang 2012).

Not only do fibromyalgia muscles use fuel inefficiently, but ongoing tension makes them burn through it quickly. Imagine constantly idling that car with bad mileage. The combination of *constant* and *inefficient* use of muscle energy makes you burn nutrients faster than they can be replaced and builds up painful waste products like lactic acid. Even at rest, fibromyalgia muscles show the level of lactic acid you would expect in someone who has run a 5K race (Gerdle 2010). Nonstop muscle tension is equivalent to nonstop exercise. No wonder we're tired and our muscles hurt! This energy imbalance can be repaired with extra nutrients that improve the muscles' ability to use fuel, in addition to reducing the tension that is overworking the muscles.

Generalized Inflammation in Fibromyalgia

The chain reaction triggered by a hyperactive stress response also leads to body-wide, generalized inflammation. This low-grade inflammation results in feeling achy and flulike, and contributes to fatigue and muscle pain. Deep-sleep deprivation increases levels of inflammatory chemicals in the body and leads to a reduced ability to fight off infection (Lentz 1999; Haack 2007). In a vicious cycle, chronic infections also produce inflammatory chemicals. Another result of the stress response is a "leaky gut," in which some food particles may enter the bloodstream and cause sensitivity-related inflammation. Thus, to reduce inflammation we must improve deep sleep and treat it at the source: hidden infections and food sensitivities.

Turning Up the Pain Volume

Chemicals secreted by the fight-or-flight nerves irritate pain-sensing nerves (the nociceptors) into sending louder signals, and in fibromyalgia they become exceptionally loud (Sato 1991; Ghilardi 2012; Longo 2013; Serra 2013). The overactivity of the nociceptors overwhelms the brain and spinal cord's ability to process those signals. This results in hypersensitivity to pain, also called central sensitization (because the *central* nervous system has become more *sensitive* to pain). Studies have shown three times more substance P, a chemical that is important in the transmission of pain signals, in the spinal fluid of fibromyalgia patients compared to healthy controls (Russell 1994; Petersel 2011). To reduce pain in fibromyalgia we need to calm the hypersensitive neurons in the spinal cord and improve the brain's ability to filter out the noise.

In addition to learning how to activate a relaxation response and improve deep sleep, my four R's treatment approach will give you the tools you need to lessen muscle tightness, improve muscle energy, and restore balance to hormones and inflammation. And you will turn the volume down on pain!

CHAPTER 5

Helping Your Doctor Help You

You may not be able to find a doctor knowledgeable about fibromyalgia, but with this book in hand all you need is one who is willing to partner with you. If you don't have a primary care provider, finding one is your first step. After you've established a relationship, ask if she'd be willing to work with you on a treatment plan. Although some specialists like rheumatologists will diagnose fibromyalgia, almost all ongoing care is performed by primary care providers. But let me remind you that the average provider sees twenty patients a day for fifteen minutes each. So you may only be able to cover one topic, or part of a topic, at each appointment. Ask whether you can set up a series of office visits to discuss various aspects of fibromyalgia management, and also if any longer appointment times are available. Some doctors will allow thirty-minute or longer visits for patients with complex issues.

FAQ: What does "health care provider" mean?

Many primary care providers are not physicians, but instead are nurse practitioners or physician assistants. When I say "doctor" what I really mean is "health care provider" (HCP), a more general term that includes medical doctors (MDs), doctors of osteopathy (DOs), family nurse practitioners (FNPs), and physician assistants (PAs).

Sample Language to Use for Partnering with Your Health Care Provider

- "I am reading a book that helps me with self-management tools for fibromyalgia. It also has evidence-based suggestions for doctors. Is this something you would be willing to partner with me on?"
- "I know fibromyalgia is a lot to cover in one office visit, so I was hoping we could schedule monthly visits for a while to make sure we have enough time to address different aspects of my treatment."
- "Is it possible for all our visits to be extended-time visits?"

I suggest photocopying the HCP handout in the appendix and giving a copy to your provider so she can review your options and work with you on implementing them. The handout briefly describes the reasoning behind different treatments and medications, with research articles that your HCP can look up. Doctors like to provide what is called evidence-based medicine, meaning treatments that research studies have shown are effective. The goal of the HCP guide is to help your provider understand the scientific reasoning behind a given approach. Keep in mind that the guide is designed for medical professionals, so it may be in medicalese, with information that I know a doctor will be specifically looking for.

FAQ: How can I read the articles that you reference?

If you are interested in reading or printing an article mentioned in this book, first find the complete listing in the reference section at the end of the book. Then go online to www.pubmed.gov, a database maintained by the United States National Library of Medicine that indexes most published research articles. The easiest way to search this database is to enter the PubMed PMID, the eight-digit number that identifies a specific article and can be found at the end of most references. The PMID will pull up an abstract, or summary, of the article. If you don't have Internet access, go to or call your nearest medical school library for help.

The HCP guide is designed for Western-trained medical professionals and does not incorporate alternative medicine. Conventional HCPs have different comfort levels with unorthodox approaches and experiences that may make them unwilling to prescribe certain medications or treatment regimens; it can even be risky for them to go against mainstream medical thinking. This is why I have also specified which topics are best addressed with an alternative medicine provider. The most qualified ones are naturopathic physicians (NDs), who undergo four years of training in holistic medicine, generally under a separate licensing board. Naturopaths are even trained to prescribe drugs, although they emphasize natural healing agents.

Conventional doctors with an integrative or holistic approach are a great option to help integrate both perspectives into your care. Integrative practitioners, like myself, use a combination of what is typically referred to as conventional medicine (i.e., what is taught in U.S. medical schools) and alternative medicine (i.e., forms of treatment or medicine that are not). A newer approach, called functional medicine, expands on the integrative approach by looking at the interactions among genetic, environmental, and lifestyle factors that affect health.

Use a Scientific Approach

It is important to be patient and to take a scientific approach to making changes. This means implementing only one or two at a time to better evaluate whether a treatment is helping you. You also need a way to track your progress, and an easy way to do that is to use a short questionnaire I developed for my clinic, which is derived from the Fibromyalgia Impact Questionnaire used in research studies. The seven-question survey asks you to rate the impact of fibromyalgia on your ability to do work (including housework), levels of pain and tenderness, fatigue, poor memory, depression, and quality of sleep. A printable version is available at www.fibromanual.com. I suggest filling it out once a week and bringing it to your doctor to review your progress over time and gauge your response to treatments.

Another option is to rate your daily pain, fatigue, and fibrofog on a scale of 0 to 10 and record it on a calendar, a journal, or your phone. You can also find smartphone apps designed to track symptoms. Remember, doctors love data! It's like someone with diabetes bringing in logs of blood sugar readings for their HCP to evaluate and use to make treatment changes. Bringing clear and concise information to your HCP will help her make good decisions on your behalf. It's also helpful for you to know which regimens are helping you and which aren't. Human memory is best at remembering the immediate past and tends to be clouded by what we are experiencing right now. When you are dealing with poor memory from fibrofog it can be near impossible to recall how you were feeling yesterday, let alone two weeks ago. Tracking your symptoms will help you and your HCP more quickly determine what works for you.

Other Keys to Partnering with Your Doctor

The American health care system is fragmented and dysfunctional. Doctors feel this crunch, especially primary care providers, many of whom see more than twenty patients a day. In an ideal world, health care providers would be able to easily access all their patients' data. But most providers don't have an easy way to communicate with or see diagnostic testing ordered by other health care providers and specialists involved in their patients' care. Ideally every X-ray, MRI, or lab test ordered by a specialist would also be sent to the primary care provider, who could then act as the data hub and direct the patient's overall care. But with the caseload that most practices see, this critical contact falls through the cracks. It is a classic case of the left hand not knowing what the right hand is doing.

Try to make your health care provider's job as easy as possible by providing her with as much of your medical information as you can, and she'll be able to avoid repeating labs and trying prescriptions that haven't worked in the past. I suggest that patients always request that a copy of any lab result, diagnostic test, sleep study, or specialist report be sent to them *and* their primary care provider. This ensures that she will have the information needed to make the most of your time at each appointment and get you on the right road sooner. I recommend that patients keep all their medical records in a designated file or notebook to take along if they have to establish care with a new health care provider. Finally, make sure to get the mammogram, colonoscopy, or any other screening tests that your doctor recommends. As a former primary care physician, I can tell you that doctors are judged (and compensated) by how many preventative services their patients complete. If your doctor has to spend valuable time and energy trying to convince you to get these tests done, that's time in which she won't be able to work with you on fibromyalgia.

Helping Your Health Care Provider to Help You

- Only focus on one or two topics in each office visit.
- Ask for extended visits each time.
- Write down non-urgent questions and try to ask them only during office visits, not over phone calls or e-mail.
- Consider setting up monthly or bimonthly visits.
- Bring copies of any new lab tests, imaging tests, or specialist reports to your appointments.
- Track your symptoms.
- Make only one change at a time.
- Do all screening/preventative tests recommended by your HCP.

Chapter Resources

- The Academy of Integrative Health & Medicine website is a good resource for finding HCPs who practice integrative medicine: www.aihm.org.
- To find a health care provider trained in functional medicine, go to the website of the Institute for Functional Medicine: www.functionalmedicine.org.
- Try using an app to track symptoms. Many of my patients like this one: www.chronicpainapp.com.
- The VASFIQ, a seven-question survey based on the Fibromyalgia Impact Questionnaire, is available at www.fibromanual.com.

CHAPTER 6

The Four R's of Fibromyalgia Treatment

The goal of treatment is to reduce the negative effects on the body of a chronic hyperactive stress response. Only by doing that can we improve pain, fatigue, and fibrofog. When I sit down with a patient to determine a treatment plan, I lay out four critical steps, the benefits of each building on the last.

The first step provides the foundation for everything else: **Rest,** giving the body a reprieve from the constant pummeling of a hyperactive stress response by enlisting a relaxation response. Despite our best efforts, once we fall asleep the fibromyalgia brain's hypervigilance again takes over and causes light, interrupted sleep, wreaking havoc on the body. Specific combinations of medications and supplements can help override that stress response and encourage deep sleep, and this is where I see the greatest improvement in fatigue and pain. This is also the step in which patients have to work most closely with their health care provider to achieve discernible results. Restoration of deep sleep allows the body to obtain as much benefit as possible from treatments such as exercise or bodywork.

Once the foundation of **Rest** is in place, we work on **Repair,** both structural and nutritional. The chronic stress response weakens the body's ability to break down and absorb nutrients, so repairing digestion is key. Structurally, the fascia and muscles are tight and "stuck." Treatment must be directed at un-sticking those tight and inflamed areas. Together, gentle exercise and manual therapy will help repair function and reduce pain in the muscles and fascia.

The next step is to **Rebalance** the problems in energy pro-duction, hormones, and inflammation. A body under chronic stress does not produce energy efficiently, so the energy-producing mitochondria need to be supported with targeted supplements. Food sensitivities and chronic infections may need to be treated as well. Burnt-out adrenal glands often need extra support to bring them back into balance. In some patients thyroid and sex hormones must be addressed. It is also essential to treat any mood disorders to regain emotional equilibrium.

Making your way through Rest, Repair, and Rebalance will result in significant improvement. In the final step, we then **Reduce** any remaining pain, fatigue, or fibrofog with targeted medications and therapies.

The Four R's of Fibromyalgia Treatment

Step 1: **Rest.** Calm the hyperactive stress response and increase deep sleep.

Step 2: **Repair.** Improve digestion and function of the muscles and fascia.

Step 3: **Rebalance.** Balance energy production, hormones, inflammation, and mood.

Step 4: **Reduce.** Treat any residual symptoms of pain, fatigue, or fibrofog.

Individualizing Treatment Regimens

Since every person with fibromyalgia is unique, there is no one size-fits-all plan. In my experience, everyone needs the core therapies in Rest and Repair, especially medication and supplements to increase deep sleep. Rest is the foundational, crucial step because reducing the stress response and improving sleep has so many positive effects on all the symptoms of fibromyalgia. Repairing digestion and treating the fascia with exercise and manual therapy is also vital. After that, patients may only need to work on a few Rebalancing and Reducing treatments, depending on their unique symptoms.

I've listed many options within each step so that you can find the ones that work the best for you. Try not to get overwhelmed as you learn about the different therapies, and remember that you don't have to do everything. Often a treatment that helps one symptom will have a positive effect on others as well, so you get a lot of two-for-one deals. For example, myofascial release therapy helps pain and reduces the stress response. Reducing inflammation levels alleviates pain and fibrofog. Each step builds on the last, and as you progress through them, you will have fewer and fewer symptoms.

Certain treatments do tend to work well for most patients, and I've highlighted those as the good places to start. Remember to try only one new medication or regimen at a time, to see what effect it has for you. Track your progress by recording your symptoms and keep in touch with your HCP at monthly visits. Reread chapter 5 to remind yourself how to optimize your partnership with your HCP and the best ways to monitor your health.

As you read the examples of patients from my practice you will see the different ways that treatments can be combined. You will notice some common features, particularly that each patient follows a regimen to increase deep sleep. As we delve into more detail later, you'll meet these patients again.

Julie is a thirty-year-old graduate student whose fatigue from fibromyalgia got so bad she had to drop out of school. After she started treatment for obstructive sleep apnea, her fatigue started to lessen. A pregabalin (Lyrica) prescription to improve sleep quality gave her even more energy. She got further pain reduction with myofascial release and was able to return to school within a year of starting treatment.

Linda is fifty-five years old and has fibromyalgia triggered by Lyme disease. With extensive antibiotic treatment over several years overseen by a naturopath, her Lyme symptoms improved, but she was left with severe muscle pain. Her sleep quality recovered with tizanidine (Zanaflex) and zolpidem (Ambien), but she was on high doses of morphine and still struggling with pain. She started eating a Paleo-type diet (low carbohydrate, no dairy, high protein), which helped her pain significantly. The addition of a low dose of propranolol, a medication that blocks some of the effects of the fight-or-flight nerves, reduced her pain even further. We were then able to lower her morphine dosage.

Debra is a forty-seven-year-old counselor who found that the addition of GABA supplement and amitriptyline improved her sleep, but pain management was still a struggle because she didn't tolerate any pain medications. She started attending a mindfulness-based stress reduction class and doing gentle yoga, which helped manage her pain levels more successfully. We found she could tolerate a topical anti-inflammatory cream that relieved pain during flares, and the addition of digestive enzymes and probiotic supplements reduced her irritable bowel symptoms.

Steve is a fifty-eight-year-old veteran with pain from osteoarthritis and fibromyalgia. Although he struggled with pain, fibrofog was the symptom that interfered with his life the most. At our initial office visit his wife had to constantly remind him to stay on track in the conversation. Steve's sleep was disturbed by nightmares, which is very common in veterans and others with post-traumatic stress disorder. I prescribed prazosin, which stopped his nightmares and improved his sleep quality. His fibrofog dramatically improved after the addition of memantine (Namenda), a medication that enhances brain functioning and is used to treat Alzheimer's. He was able to stay focused in conversation and told me, "I feel like I have my brain back."

Maureen is a retired nurse in her sixties who has struggled with fibromyalgia for over twenty years. Taking gabapentin at bedtime made a huge difference in her fatigue and pain levels. She had tried and failed multiple exercise regimens and reported that they all aggravated her pain. After she started doing a gentle but complete warm-up (see page 98) before walking on a treadmill she could finally exercise without causing a flare-up. For further pain reduction she uses a topical marijuana salve applied to her neck and shoulders.

Pam is a forty-four-year-old self-described "Diet Coke addict" who had been taking high-dose daily tramadol for years. Over time, it stopped giving her much relief. Once she cut out soda and began avoiding all artificial sweeteners, her pain decreased to the point that she no longer required daily tramadol and could take it just as needed for pain. A combination of trazodone and gabapentin improved her quality of sleep and fatigue levels.

Michelle is a thirty-nine-year-old single mother of three who first came to me while going through a long, stressful divorce and legal battle. She had hypothyroidism in addition to fibromyalgia and was struggling with profound fatigue. Although her thyroid lab indicated adequate hormone levels, she had many symptoms of low thyroid, including hair loss and edema. I adjusted her thyroid regimen, but her fatigue did not improve until we supported her adrenals with a short course of hydrocortisone and supplements. Cyclobenzaprine and magnesium helped get her sleep back on track, and for pain flares she takes tramadol as needed and gets trigger point injections into her neck and shoulder muscles.

Core Supplements for Fibromyalgia

As you read through the treatment chapters, you will learn about various supplements that can help with specific symptoms of fibromyalgia. But you don't have to take every one I mention. In fact, the key here is to keep it simple. Focus on those that have scientific support, or that you personally find helpful. I often see patients struggling to keep up with complicated and expensive supplement regimens, and I work with them to streamline it down to the essentials.

The core, long-term supplements that I have all of my patients take are those that are well known to support healthy functioning of the nervous system and mitochondria, including B vitamins, fish oil, vitamin D, and magnesium. I also recommend probiotics and digestive enzymes to aid in digestion and prevent irritable bowel syndrome. In the chapters to come, you will learn more about why I recommend these specific supplements and the recommended dosages.

I also suggest optional supplements aimed at specific problems that may only be needed for a short period of time, such as leaky gut repair or adrenal burnout treatment. I personally can't keep up with any regimen that involves more than six different pills a day, so I try to keep it simple for my patients too.

Core Fibromyalgia Supplements

Activated B vitamins (see page 126)
Vitamin D (see page 127)
Fish oil (see page 141)
Magnesium (see page 76)
Probiotics (see page 92)
Digestive enzymes (see page 88)

The Four R's Journey

When I see a new patient, I first make sure that fibromyalgia is the correct diagnosis. Many illnesses can mimic fibromyalgia, so it's important to see a health care provider to confirm the diagnosis. If your primary care provider does not feel comfortable or have the expertise to make that call, ask for referral to a rheumatologist, pain specialist, or neurologist.

Once we have a confirmed diagnosis, my patients participate in an intensive education program on self-treatment of the fascia, inducing a relaxation response, and learning how to exercise. They learn much of the information outlined in the Rest and Repair sections of this book, which is of course very important. But the biggest benefit is often the mutual support from the other students. I heard a speaker say once that many people with fibromyalgia end up "spiritually and emotionally" bankrupt, and I could not agree more. Many patients have had to fight against family, doctors, and employers not understanding their condition for so long that they are bitter and weary. Real emotional healing can come from the support that only someone who knows exactly how you feel can give. I strongly encourage you to seek out other people with fibromyalgia. The National Fibromyalgia & Chronic Pain Association and the National Fibromyalgia Association can provide help and connect you with local support groups. There is also an active fibromyalgia Facebook community. I have included my own story and the stories of my patients in this book because I want you to know that you are not alone in this journey.

Making any change can be hard. It is much, much harder when you feel exhausted and in pain. When people who don't have fibromyalgia ask me how it feels, I tell them to imagine the last time they had a bad flu, then to picture going shopping, cooking, or exercising while feeling like that.

The four R's treatment program you are embarking on does require you to make some adjustments to how you eat, move, and sleep. It's easy to feel overwhelmed by the number of things you have to do. My advice is to start at the beginning and go one step at a time. Read through the whole treatment section if you want, but then go back and closely reread the Rest section. The order of these chapters is intentional—each builds on the last—so don't skip around in these first two steps. You'll need around three to four months to complete Rest and Repair. So for the next month or two focus *only* on the three Rest chapters. Every day try to do something to activate the relaxation response. Make an appointment with your doctor to talk about sleep. Only once you have made some progress with getting deep sleep, move on to Repair and spend the next one to two months strengthening digestion and doing gentle exercise and fascia treatment. Then you can either continue reading each chapter in order, or skip around to those parts of Rebalance and Reduce that you feel will be most helpful.

Be patient with yourself, and know that you don't have to do it all. Just *start*. Each step that you complete will help you feel better, and will make it easier to tackle the next one. To borrow from Alcoholics Anonymous, "work the program and the program will work."

Chapter Resources

- National Fibromyalgia & Chronic Pain Association, www .fmcpaware.org and www.fibroandpain.org.
- National Fibromyalgia Association, www.fmaware.org.

CHAPTER 7

Rest: Taming the Hyperactive
Stress Response

In chapters 3 and 4, you learned how fibromyalgia symptoms stem from a hyperactive stress response. The foundation of treatment is taking action on a daily basis to instead activate the opposite reaction: the relaxation response. The relaxation response stimulates the rest-and-digest nerves that have positive effects on the body.

As you recall, alarm signals sent out by the hypothalamus cause the hyperactive stress response to constantly rouse our fight-or-flight nerves, resulting in muscle tension, pain, and inefficient energy use. It also interferes with sleep, resulting in light, non-restful sleep. So it stands to reason that if we could find a way to reset the hypothalamus—to turn off the alarm—we would be able to reverse fibromyalgia. So far we don't have a way to do this, but we can hit the snooze bar and give our body a break. The body's snooze bar is the relaxation response, and the more you press it, the more benefit you will see. So, how do we create a relaxation response?

Calling On the Relaxation Response

Let's try an experiment. Stop reading for a moment and tell your body to relax. Nothing happened, right? Now take three slow deep breaths, feeling the air move in through your nose, opening up your chest, and allow the air to leak slowly back out. Check in with your body. Can you feel that your muscles are less tense and your jaw is not as clenched? You just activated your relaxation response! What was the difference? Why can't you just command your body to relax and have it obey?

The parts of the brain that control stress and relaxation are not under the control of the thinking brain. Remember, the hypothalamus and the brain stem are within the deep primal area of the brain that functions on autopilot and does not respond to commands from the conscious mind. In fact, they are busy controlling your heart rate, blood pressure, and digestion while your thinking brain reads this book.

You did not think your way into a hyperactive stress response, and you can't think your way out of it. By the same token, you can't think your way into relaxation. Instead, you must use your body to make the brain relax.

Ways to Trigger a Relaxation Response

- Deep slow belly breaths
- Gentle exercise
- Guided relaxation
- Meditation/mindfulness practices
- Biofeedback therapy
- Cranial electrotherapy stimulation (CES)
- Craniosacral therapy
- Myofascial release therapy

- Acupuncture
- Flotation tanks
- Gargling
- Singing
- Doing something that gives you joy
- Transdermal magnesium

Making Your Brain Stem Listen to You

Your brain stem only listens to signals from the body, not from the thinking parts of the brain. So you must intentionally change the message that your body is sending, and the best way to do that is by controlling your breathing. Breathing is the only bodily function that we do both consciously and unconsciously. Breath control represents a unique overlap of our thinking brain and our autopilot brain. Slow, deep breaths that expand your belly are especially powerful at eliciting a relaxation response, so that's the simplest and best way to reduce stress.

It may be helpful to set aside a daily designated relaxation time: lie in a comfortable place and take ten deep slow breaths. In his seminal 1975 book *The Relaxation Response,* Dr. Herbert Benson, a pioneering mind-body researcher, describes various techniques: in addition to slowing your breathing, you can also try gentle exercise, yoga, tai chi, and warm-water pool therapy. In chapter 11, you will learn how to exercise in the right way for fibromyalgia.

Some people also find relief through meditation and guided muscle relaxation. Mindfulness meditation, the efficacy of which has been extensively studied, involves increasing your awareness and observation of your breath, thoughts, and bodily sensations in order to promote relaxation. Mindfulness-based stress reduction (MBSR) classes teach this technique over six to eight weeks. My patient Debra, whom you met in the last chapter, found that the skills she learned in this class were key to taming her stress response.

FAQ: Do I have to meditate?

Meditation doesn't work for everyone. I personally have not had much success with meditation on its own. (In fact, whenever I try to just "observe my breath," I end up almost hyperventilating.) Some people do better practicing deep breathing and increased body awareness in combination with movement, like yoga or tai chi. I find that yoga, which combines deep breathing with movement and stretching, helps me relax most easily. But many people find relief through meditation, and there are lots of different techniques out there—try a few and see if you find a good match. Guided relaxation and meditation apps for smartphones allow you to practice wherever you are.

Biofeedback therapy, which promotes body awareness, is a more high-tech way to induce relaxation. Monitors are placed on your muscles so you can see where they are tightest and practice relaxing those areas—while you watch in real time. They also measure your pulse and encourage you to slow it down with deep breathing and visualizations. If you find a physical or occupational therapist knowledgeable about biofeedback, they may even be able to set you up with tools at home.

The vagus nerve is the major highway for the rest-and-digest nerves, and it controls the back of the throat, so any activity that stimulates the vagus nerve will also induce relaxation. Gently gagging yourself with your toothbrush does it, as does gargling. Loud singing will also do the trick (and is an excellent way to relax if it gives you joy, too!).

Another therapy that has been shown to reduce cortisol levels, muscle tension, and pain, and induce relaxation is called reduced environmental stimulation therapy (REST), in which you float in a shallow warm pool about the size of a large bed, enclosed in a lightproof, soundproof tank that drastically reduces sensory input (van Dierendonck 2005). The water is saturated with about a thousand pounds of Epsom salt (magnesium sulfate) to make it heavy and enable easy floating. Magnesium also promotes muscle relaxation. It's like taking a bath while floating like a cork on the surface of the water. One of my patients told me it was the most effective tool she had found for fibromyalgia relief. In the float tank she is able to completely relax, allowing her to unlock painful and tight areas of muscle.

Many societies around the world have long histories of bathing in natural hot springs rich in minerals to improve health. The custom is finally catching on in the United States, with "float houses" springing up in larger cities. It's a unique experience; it feels like, I imagine, floating in space. Without the effect of gravity on your joints and muscles, there is less input to the pain-sensing nerves, resulting in less pain. In the float tank and for a few days after, my pain is decreased, my muscles feel looser, and my body is calmer. If you can't access flotation therapy, you can simulate its effects at home by taking a bath with as much Epsom salt as you can get to dissolve. Then turn off the lights and reduce noise as much as possible. You won't float unless you have a huge bathtub (and a thousand pounds of salt), but you will still get the relaxing benefits of magnesium absorbed through your skin.

Transdermal Magnesium

Magnesium is the relaxation mineral: it has calming effects on the brain, nerves, and muscles. And what mineral is nearly everyone with fibromyalgia deficient in? You guessed it! Most of the body's magnesium is stored inside cells, so to gauge levels accurately, we need to check there. When scientists have analyzed the levels of magnesium inside red blood cells in fibromyalgia patients, they are consistently low (Eisinger 1994). Hair testing analysis has also confirmed lower-than-average levels (Kim 2011). In one study, magnesium oral supplementation was shown to improve symptoms (Bagis 2013). But there are a few challenges with taking this mineral orally. It acts as a laxative (you may have heard of milk of magnesia, one of the strongest laxatives there is), and we don't absorb it very efficiently through our intestines. Oral magnesium supplements help support healthy adrenal function and boost energy production (see chapters 13 and 15 for more information), but to trigger a relaxation response, you need to get the high doses that can only be attained by letting your skin and muscles soak it up.

We absorb magnesium better through our skin than through our intestines, so a transdermal application is an effective way to trigger relaxation. You may bathe in Epsom salt or rub magnesium oil or lotion on your feet and legs before bed, which guides the body into deeper sleep and acts as natural relaxant to tight muscles. Be careful, though, as magnesium can be a bit abrasive to the skin, so if you have an open cut don't use it on that area—it will sting. The creams and lotions are milder and gentler on the skin than the oils, but contain less magnesium.

Manual Therapies

There are two types of manual therapy that can induce a relaxation response: craniosacral, and myofascial release. Craniosacral therapy developed from the osteopathic medical tradition in which a therapist gently manipulates the base of the skull and near the tailbone with the hands. The fluid around the brain and spinal cord, called the cerebrospinal fluid, has rhythmic pulsations, and that subtle wavelike motion acts like a pump to clear toxins and waste products from the brain. This has been documented on MRI imaging (Feinberg 1987). These pulsations can be manually interpreted—and altered—by a trained therapist. Because the nerves of the parasympathetic (rest-and-digest) nervous system exit the spinal cord at the top near the base of the skull (cranium) and at the bottom near the tailbone (sacrum), gentle manipulation of fluid in those areas stimulates relaxation.

I have experienced craniosacral therapy as part of a massage or myofascial release session, and find it incredibly calming. Usually, the base of my skull is resting on the therapist's hands, and after a few slight movements I start to feel very sleepy and heavy, like slipping into a hot bath. There is also a wonderful device called the CranioCradle that you can use at home to simulate craniosacral therapy. You rest the back of your head on its soft foam, which puts light stimulating pressure on the base of your skull, and with a few deep slow breaths your body comes to a place of deep relaxation. It also softens the tight fascia in the back of the neck, which can bring pain relief.

Myofascial release is a manual therapy that reduces tension in the fascia, the connective tissue around muscles. You will learn more about using this therapy to reduce fibromyalgia pain, but it also induces a relaxation response in the body. The fascia contains many fight-or-flight nerve endings, and gentle sustained pressure of myofascial release calms them and lowers their activity (Tanaka 1977). A study found reduced signals from fight-or-flight nerves for twenty-four hours after this therapy was applied to the pelvic fascia (Cottingham 1988). Fascial stretching sends a "calm down" message through the fight-or-flight nerves back up to the brain stem, turning down fight-or-flight and turning up rest-and-digest, with lingering relaxation effects. You can also self-administer myofascial release, which you will learn more about in the Repair section.

Acupuncture

Many patients report great results from acupuncture, which brain monitoring studies show can stimulate the relaxation response. One study found that acupuncture increased activity of the rest-and-digest nerves during treatment and for sixty minutes afterward (Haker 2000; Sakai 2007). Acupuncture has even been shown to lower the signals from fight-or-flight nerves in rats (Imai 2009). The fact that acupuncture works on both humans and lab rats means that it is not a placebo response (in which patients feel better after a treatment due to their expectation that it is going to help): a lab rat doesn't go into an experiment thinking that an acupuncture needle is going to benefit it!

Cranial Electrotherapy Stimulation

Another therapy that affects the brain directly is called cranial electrotherapy stimulation (CES), which uses microcurrent levels of electricity transmitted between electrodes placed on each ear. The level of electricity is so low that it is generally not detectable to the user. This technique is thought to directly activate the parasympathetic (rest-and-digest) nervous system where it leaves the brain stem. It was developed in the Soviet Union in the 1950s as a sleep inducer and was heavily researched in the United States in the 1970s as a treatment for anxiety. One of my patients called it "meditation without all the work." CES has been shown to induce a sense of calm or clearheadedness; even a single session may reduce anxiety and muscle tension as effectively as a session of guided relaxation. Two different, well-designed placebo-controlled studies demon-strated reduction in pain and anxiety symptoms in fibromyal-gia (Lichtbroun 2001; Cork 2004).

I tried using CES therapy for about a month, for thirty min-utes a day. At higher settings it gave me a headache and I could feel a prickly sensation in my ears. But at the lowest setting (the level used in studies because it is below the threshold of sensa-tion), I found it very relaxing, and it helped me fall asleep more quickly at night. The biggest challenge is financial; the devices are expensive. Some companies will let you rent one, and health insurance may cover part of the cost with a prescription.

Finding Your Relaxation Triggers

Since we don't consciously control the stress response, we can't "think" it away. But we can use our body to signal our brain that it's time to relax. I encourage you to experiment and find what works the best for you. Regardless of the method you use, it is essential to guide your body there as often as you can. In fibro-myalgia, daily effort must be made to reduce the stress response and its negative effects on the body. Practicing these techniques regularly can help with every aspect of the chain reaction caused by a hyperactive stress response.

Try not to be overwhelmed by all the different therapies we just learned about, because you always have the simplest and most effective tool with you—your own breath. Every time you become aware of the effects of stress in your body such as mus-cle tightness or clenching, remind yourself to take a few slow, deep breaths. I find it helpful to consciously try to relax my pel-vic and jaw muscles as I breathe. Others think about breathing into their hips or another tense body part.

Remember that efforts to trigger the relaxation response will reduce the negative effects of a hyperactive stress re-sponse and are the foundation of treating fibromyalgia.

To Do Yourself

- Visit www.heartmath.com for more information on home biofeedback therapy.
- Learn more about craniosacral therapy at www.upledger .com.
- Find a tool to give yourself craniosacral therapy at www .craniocradle.com. The site has instructional videos and purchasing information (it costs around $35).
- Learn more about myofascial release and find a local therapist at www.myofascialrelease.com.
- Get a fun and easy meditation app at www.headspace.com.
- Search online to find mindfulness-based stress reduction (MBSR) classes in your area.
- Learn about flotation therapy for fibromyalgia at www .fibromyalgiaflotationproject.com.
- Order transdermal magnesium at www.ancient-minerals .com.

To Discuss with Your Health Care Provider

- Ask about a prescription for cranial electrotherapy stimulation (CES). The best-studied device is made by a company called Alpha-Stim (www.alpha-stim.com).
- Request a referral to a physical or occupational therapist who does biofeedback.

CHAPTER 8

Rest: Fixing Fibromyalgia Sleep

*In fibromyalgia all treatments are geared toward
helping people sleep better. If we can improve their
sleep, patients will get better.*
—DR. STEVEN BERNEY, CHIEF OF RHEUMATOLOGY
AT TEMPLE UNIVERSITY (DAVIS N.D.)

Treating sleep is the key to treating fibromyalgia, and where I see the most benefit in reducing pain, fatigue, and brain fog. Sleep must always be improved before any other treatment will work, so it's the first step to address with your HCP. Unfortunately, many doctors, even sleep specialists, are not aware of the connection. But fibromyalgia is primarily a sleep disorder, a state of chronic deep-sleep deprivation. Studies have consistently demonstrated that patients experience inadequate deep sleep that is frequently interrupted by "wakeful" brain waves. This leads to the fatigue, muscle pain, and foggy thinking characteristic of the condition.

Sleep Problems Seen in Fibromyalgia

- Not enough deep sleep
- Choppy deep sleep
- Multiple "microawakenings"
- Abnormal "awake" brain waves

Because most doctors are unaware of this research, they are also not knowledgeable about how to improve fibromyalgia sleep. By far the most effective medication is sodium oxybate (Xyrem), which induces deep sleep (Staud 2011). Unfortunately, it was denied FDA approval in 2010 due to the risk of illicit usage, and the movement to research and treat sleep in fibromyalgia disappeared. In the next chapter you will learn about combinations of currently available medications that simulate what Xyrem does for the sleeping brain. But first we need to eliminate any other problems that may be interfering with sleep quality. And to do that, we need to understand a little more about both normal healthy sleep and the abnormal sleep we see in fibromyalgia.

Normal Sleep

Normal human sleep consists of a regular pattern of different cycles: light sleep, deep sleep, and dreaming sleep (also called REM or rapid eye movement sleep). These stages are distinguished by different types of brain activity. In deep sleep, brain waves (reflecting electrical activity in the brain) are slow; in light sleep they are a little faster. During dreaming sleep, brain waves are very fast and accompanied by eye movements—that's why it's also called rapid eye movement sleep. We spend more time in deep sleep earlier in the night, and more time in dreaming sleep toward the morning.

Deep sleep is the most important of these three phases—it's what makes you feel rested the next day. It is when your tissues—especially muscles—undergo healing and repair. We spend more time in deep sleep after exercise to repair muscle tissue. Most growth hormone secretion occurs during this stage, of which adequate amounts are vital for proper muscle and tissue repair. Finally, deep sleep is the time when toxic waste products are cleared from the brain (Xie 2013). With too little deep sleep, we feel fatigued, our muscles ache, and our brains are foggy. Sounds familiar, doesn't it?

Light sleep	Deep sleep	REM sleep
• Occurs during 55 percent of night • Involves medium brain waves • Easy to be awoken	• Occurs during 20 percent of night • Involves very slow brain waves • No dreaming • Growth hormone released • Muscle tissue repair occurs • Difficult to be awoken	• Occurs during 25 percent of night • Involves fast brain waves • Dreaming • Eyes dart back and forth • Easy to be awoken

Fibromyalgia Sleep

In fibromyalgia, normal sleep patterns are disrupted and sleep is of very poor quality: light, choppy, and lacking the normal periods of "delta wave" or deep sleep (Moldofsky 2008). Studies consistently show that patients with fibromyalgia don't spend much time in deep sleep, and the deep sleep they do get is interrupted by fast "wakeful" brain waves (alpha waves) that are normally only seen in the awake brain, a phenomenon called "alpha-wave intrusion" (Branco 1994).

Most sleep studies ordered by doctors attempt only to diagnose sleep apnea and thus don't report the number of alpha intrusions, which must be done by hand and is labor intensive. There is also no consistent way to document the frequency of alpha waves. But exciting new research done by Dr. Victor Rosenfeld, a sleep physician, may change that. He has developed a specialized computer program to quickly analyze a sleep study by counting the alpha waves (awake) compared to delta (deep sleep) waves, which gives a delta-alpha ratio. He has found that a low delta-alpha score (a disproportionate amount of alpha waves compared to delta waves) consistently occurs in patients with fibromyalgia (Rosenfeld 2015). If his work is confirmed in larger studies, a low delta-alpha ratio may eventually be used as an objective marker for diagnosis of fibromyalgia. As you know, the current diagnostic criteria rely on clinical markers alone, and we need to find a consistent benchmark to really advance research and treatment.

The cause of alpha intrusion seems to be the stress response system, which in a healthy person is quiet at night, but in fibromyalgia remains continually active (Kooh 2003). The brain won't allow itself to fully sink into deep sleep because it's trying to remain awake in order to fight off a threat by "sleeping with one eye open."

Deep sleep in fibromyalgia also shows a choppy pattern that is interrupted by frequent microawakenings. In healthy sleep, the brain stays in deep sleep for a period of time, usually twenty or thirty minutes, before cycling back to a lighter stage. In contrast, in fibromyalgia the brain jumps back and forth from deep to light sleep, often staying in deep sleep for less than a minute, so the brain and body never get the full benefit of prolonged deep sleep.

The constant state of sleep deprivation leaves the brain and

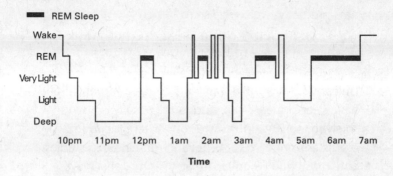

Normal sleep pattern.

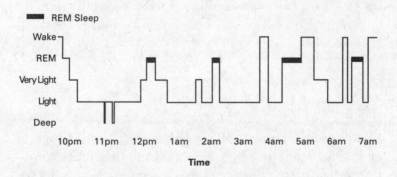

Typical fibromyalgia sleep pattern.

body starving for deep sleep—the most "nutritious" form of sleep, the "broccoli" of sleep. Light sleep is like Twinkies: calories but no nutritional value. Fibromyalgia muscles are surviving on Twinkies and don't get enough of the good stuff, which leads to pain. Dr. Harvey Moldofsky, one of the first researchers to study fibromyalgia sleep, proposed back in 1975 that it should be considered a "non-restorative sleep syndrome." He was able to induce fibromyalgia symptoms of muscle pain and fatigue in healthy college students after a few nights of deep-sleep deprivation, which went away after they resumed normal sleep (Moldofsky 1975).

FAQ: Should I get a sleep study to look for alpha intrusions?

Unless you or your doctor are concerned you might have sleep apnea, sleep studies are usually not worth it solely to look for alpha intrusions. There is currently no consistent standard for reporting data in sleep studies, and most don't comment at all on alpha waves. If delta-alpha ratios were adopted and consistently reported in sleep studies based on Dr. Rosenfeld's analysis, then I would recommend that everyone with fibromyalgia get a sleep study to confirm the diagnosis.

Fixing Fibromyalgia Sleep

So how do we increase the time spent in deep sleep and get rid of wakeful brain waves? First, we find and treat related problems such as obstructive sleep apnea and restless legs syndrome. Next, we eliminate habits and medications that are harming sleep quality. Finally, we add medications that increase the amount of time spent in deep sleep (covered in greater depth in chapter 9).

How to Fix Fibromyalgia Sleep

- Find and treat other sleep disorders.
- Eliminate medications that are harming sleep quality.
- Improve sleep habits.
- Use medications that promote deep sleep.

Evaluate and Treat Any Other Sleep Disorders

My first recommendation for fibromyalgia patients looking to improve their sleep is to make sure they don't have any other sleep disorders that may need to be treated. Half of people with fibromyalgia also have an additional disorder such as obstructive sleep apnea or restless legs syndrome that can make sleep even worse (Gold 2004; Shah 2006; Viola-Saltzman 2010).

The hormonal changes around menopause can also wreak havoc on sleep. If you are having insomnia or frequent awakenings due to night sweats, talk to your HCP about treatment, which usually includes hormone replacement therapy. Hormone replacement therapy in menopausal women has been shown to improve sleep quality (Gambacciani 2005), but you'll need to discuss the pros and cons since it is also associated with increased risk of certain cancers. In chapter 16 you will learn about other natural ways to balance your hormones and reduce the side effects of menopause.

Obstructive Sleep Apnea

Obstructive sleep apnea (OSA) is a common sleep disorder caused when the soft tissue in the back of the throat collapses and blocks the airway, stopping your breathing (apnea). This can occur hundreds of times an hour, and with each apnea the brain receives a powerful arousal signal in order to trigger a breath, resulting in fragmented and poor-quality sleep, and profound fatigue during the day. Treatment usually involves wearing a mask that pushes oxygen into your lungs to keep your airway open, called continuous positive airway pressure (CPAP).

With fibromyalgia it is extremely important to diagnose and treat any OSA, because even mild sleep apnea is a huge stimulator of the stress response. If left untreated, it will significantly worsen the already disrupted sleep patterns in fibromyalgia, and any improvement in deep sleep will be nearly impossible. Men with fibromyalgia commonly have underlying sleep apnea, so I refer all my male patients for a sleep study (Rosenfeld 2015; May 1993). I only order sleep studies for female patients who have risk factors for OSA such as obesity, smoking, or a thick neck. Julie, one of my patients you met, finally found relief from her fatigue once she learned she had OSA and started treatment.

People with sleep apnea are often unaware of the multiple awakenings/arousals they experience each night, although bed partners might note loud snoring or episodes of loud gasps for air. The only way to diagnose OSA is with a sleep study, which usually involves staying overnight in a sleep lab or hospital, during which your sleep is closely monitored. Machines register your breathing and movement, and EEG analysis of your brain waves reveals how much time you spend in each stage of sleep. Some studies can be done at home with a portable kit, but these do not give as much information and may need to be followed up with a study in the hospital or sleep lab.

FAQ: If I am diagnosed with sleep apnea, will I have to wear a breathing mask?

Very mild sleep apnea can be treated with weight loss and changing your sleeping position—the condition tends to worsen when sleeping on your back. Alternative treatments for mild cases include custom mouthpieces that shift the lower jaw forward to open up the airway. There are also small devices placed just inside the nostrils that keep your airway open by creating pressure when you exhale. Treatment for moderate or severe sleep apnea does require a breathing mask, called CPAP or BiPAP, but there are many varieties, and most people can find one that works for them.

A condition called central sleep apnea occurs when the brain "forgets" to breathe. This is most commonly seen with medications that affect the breathing regulation centers of the brain, especially in people on both benzodiazepines and opiates, so this combination should be avoided. Central sleep apnea can be diagnosed by a sleep study and is treated by changing medications, and in some cases by using CPAP or BiPAP.

Could I Have Obstructive Sleep Apnea (OSA?)

- Do you snore loudly (louder than talking or loud enough to be heard through closed doors)?
- Has anyone observed you stop breathing during your sleep?
- Has anyone ever observed you gasping or choking at night?
- Do you often wake up with a headache?
- Do you have difficulty staying awake while driving?
- Do you often fall asleep when you don't intend to (i.e., at work or in public)?
- Do you have high blood pressure?
- Do you have atrial fibrillation?
- Are you overweight?
- Is your neck circumference greater than 15.75 inches? Measure the neck circumference at a point just below the larynx (Adam's apple).
- Are you male?

If you answered yes to two or more of these questions, ask your HCP about ordering a sleep study to evaluate for sleep apnea.

Restless Legs Syndrome

Restless legs syndrome (RLS) is a neurological disorder characterized by throbbing, pulling, creeping or other unpleasant sensations in the legs and an uncontrollable, overwhelming urge to move them. Lying down and trying to relax triggers the symptoms, so most people with RLS have difficulty falling and staying asleep. RLS is fairly common in fibromyalgia, occurring in about one-third of female patients, and can be a significant cause of insomnia and sleep disruption (Viola-Saltzman 2010).

Could I Have Restless Legs Syndrome?

- Do you often get a strong urge to move your legs to relieve unpleasant sensations?
- Are the symptoms worse when you're sitting still or lying down and resting?
- Do you get temporary relief from moving your legs or walking?
- Do the symptoms start or get worse in the evening or at night?

If you answered yes to one or more of these questions, ask your HCP if you might have restless legs syndrome.

RLS is related to low levels of the brain chemical dopamine. Iron is required for production of dopamine, so people with iron deficiency anemia often have restless legs. Because of this iron-dopamine connection, if you have RLS it is important to monitor your iron levels and replace any deficiency. Testing includes a complete blood count and measuring the levels of iron and ferritin (the best way to gauge the amount of iron in your bloodstream).

In the case of RLS, however, it is not just the level of iron in your bloodstream but the amount in your brain that matters. People with normal ferritin levels can also have RLS, possibly due to low iron in the brain. One of my patients with severe RLS and normal blood iron and ferritin had her symptoms eliminated after a series of intravenous (IV) iron infusions, which is the most effective way to get iron into the brain. Not everyone with RLS needs IV iron, of course, but I saw firsthand how RLS may reflect low brain levels of iron. One study found that IV iron infusions showed significant improvement of RLS symptoms in 68 percent of the subjects without any major adverse effects (Cho 2013).

If you have RLS, I advise getting your iron and ferritin levels tested. If those levels are low, take iron supplements to get back up into normal range (ferritin levels above 50). Even for my patients with normal iron and ferritin levels, I often add an iron supplement to see if they get any improvement in their RLS symptoms. Be sure to talk with your HCP before starting iron, as your levels will need to be monitored to ensure they don't get too high.

Metanx, a prescription vitamin that contains active forms of B_6, B_{12}, and folate, has helped some of my patients with RLS, because these nutrients all increase the ability of the body to utilize iron. Other treatments include prescription medications that increase dopamine levels in the brain such as carbidopa/levodopa (Sinemet), pramipexole (Mirapex), and ropinirole (Requip). Gabapentin and pregabalin at bedtime can relieve symptoms, as can magnesium supplements. Several of my patients find benefit from applying magnesium oils and lotions to their legs just before bed.

Improve Sleep Habits to Improve Sleep Quality

After treating any sleep disorders, the next step is working with the rhythmic nature of sleep and establishing routines. Anyone who has kids knows the importance of routines, including set bedtimes and specific bedtime rituals: first bath, then brush teeth and read a story, and so on. We stick to it each night *because it works*. We also don't let them stay up late, eat candy at bedtime, or sleep with the TV blaring and lights on! But we tend not to follow these types of habits ourselves. Practicing good sleep hygiene is simply about encouraging consistent routines and avoiding factors that interfere with sleep.

Sleep Hygiene: Behaviors and Habits to Improve Sleep

Reduce caffeine. Do not consume any food, drugs, or drinks that contain caffeine or other stimulants after 2 p.m.

Do not drink alcohol or smoke within four hours of bedtime.

Do not eat a heavy meal just before bedtime.

Maintain consistent body rhythms. Create sleep patterns by going to bed at the same time and getting up at the same time every day.

Avoid napping during the day.

Create a quiet, relaxing bedroom. Try earplugs or a white noise machine if your room isn't peaceful or you sleep with a snoring partner. Make sure the bedroom is dark; buy blackout curtains if necessary. Don't use it for non-sleep activities such as working or eating. Consider buying a new bed if yours is uncomfortable.

FAQ: Should I get a Tempur-Pedic bed?

The three beds that my patients find most comfortable are memory foam/Tempur-Pedic beds, adjustable pressure beds like Sleep Number, and pillow-top mattresses. Tempur-Pedic beds are expensive, though, so using a memory foam topper for your regular mattress may be a more viable option.

Eliminate or Reduce Medications That Interfere with Deep Sleep

Finally, we have to make sure that you're not taking any medications that harm sleep quality—and unfortunately, two groups of medications commonly used to treat fibromyalgia symptoms are actually destructive to deep sleep. Opiate-based pain medications and benzodiazepines (antianxiety medications) reduce time spent in deep sleep, leading to a vicious cycle of fatigue. To improve sleep quality, eliminate these medications completely, or if that's not possible take them as early in the day as you can.

Morphine and methadone have both been shown to reduce the amount of time spent in deep sleep per night, and this partially explains why opiates have not been found very helpful long term in managing fibromyalgia pain (Dimsdale 2007; Shaw 2005). For prescriptions to be beneficial, they must be the right medications, used in the right way, as you will learn in chapter 20. I recommend taking any necessary opiates as far away from bedtime as possible to limit their negative impact.

The antianxiety medications known as benzodiazepines are often prescribed for insomnia, and while they may help you to fall asleep, sleep quality will be poor (Hindmarch 2005). In fact, benzodiazepines are my absolute last choice for treating insomnia in fibromyalgia, and in the next chapter you will learn about better options that both treat insomnia and increase the time spent in deep sleep. If you need them for anxiety, try to keep them away from sleep hours as much as possible, or check out chapter 17 for several alternatives that do not interfere with deep sleep. If you are currently taking a benzodiazepine for sleep and want to stop, make sure you talk with your HCP first to determine a tapering schedule. Ceasing benzodiazepines suddenly can cause a life-threatening withdrawal.

Benzodiazepine Medications

clonazepam (Klonopin)

lorazepam (Ativan)

diazepam (Valium)

alprazolam (Xanax)

temazepam (Restoril)

triazolam (Halcion)

Alcohol also has negative effects on sleep, so limiting intake in the several hours before bedtime is important (Feige 2006). As anyone who has lain awake for hours after having an after-dinner coffee knows, caffeine and other stimulants also have very obvious effects. Avoid caffeine after 2 p.m. since it can last for about eight hours in the body. If you take stimulants such as Adderall or Ritalin, avoid the long-acting formulations and take your last dosage no later than 2 p.m.

Strategies to Reduce Deep Sleep Interference

- Eliminate nighttime benzodiazepines and opiates.
- Avoid alcohol for four hours before bedtime.
- Avoid caffeine after 2 p.m.
- Avoid long-acting stimulant medications.

To Do Yourself

- Establish good sleep habits.
- Avoid alcohol within four hours of bedtime.
- Avoid caffeine and other stimulants after 2 p.m.

To Discuss with Your Health Care Provider

- Ask about reducing or moving any medications that interfere with sleep such as stimulants, benzodiazepines, and opiate-based pain medications.
- If you answered yes to two or more questions on the OSA questionnaire, ask about getting tested for obstructive sleep apnea.
- Ask about an alternative non-CPAP therapy for mild obstructive sleep apnea (www.proventtherapy.com).
- If you answered yes to one or more questions on the RLS questionnaire, ask about possible RLS diagnosis and treatment.
- If you want to try Metanx, a prescription nutritional supplement that can help RLS, ask your HCP about a prescription. If insurance does not cover the cost, have the prescription sent to Brand Direct Health pharmacy for a reduced cash price: www.branddirecthealth.com.

CHAPTER 9

Rest: Medications to Increase Deep Sleep

Our treatment goal here is to increase the amount of time in deep sleep not interrupted by wakeful brain waves. To do this we have to (safely!) overwhelm the arousal in the brain and push it into deep sleep. Several medications that act on different parts of the brain can help overwhelm that hyperactive stress response.

I saw firsthand the critical importance of treating sleep in fibromyalgia through my own experience with a powerful medication called sodium oxybate (Xyrem). Xyrem increases deep sleep, and multiple studies found that it reduced pain and fatigue in fibromyalgia (Staud 2011). Indeed, my symptoms improved significantly, but I was only able to take it for two months; in 2010 the FDA denied approval for its use in fibromyalgia, largely due to concerns about abuse. Its only approved use is to treat narcolepsy, a rare sleep disorder characterized by "sleep attacks" during everyday activity.

FAQ: Can I take Xyrem even though it's not FDA-approved for fibromyalgia?

Unfortunately, many doctors are unwilling to prescribe it and insurance won't cover it for fibromyalgia—and it costs thousands of dollars a month. Disappointingly, I don't think Xyrem will ever gain approval for fibromyalgia since it is chemically related to an illegal drug, GHB (gamma-hydroxybutyric acid), that has been used in some cases of date rape.

The good news is that the research on Xyrem confirmed that if we can encourage deep sleep in people with fibromyalgia, we see impressive symptom improvement. Through extensive trial and error I have found ways to simulate Xyrem's effects, but it often takes a combination of a few medications. First, we need a medication that slows brain activity. For some patients that alone may be enough. But if you're still having insomnia, we can add a sedative that causes you to fall asleep and stay asleep. The final intervention, if required, is to block the alarm signals being sent by the hyperactive stress response that continues to wake up the brain.

It can take some time to find the right combination that safely overwhelms the brain and pushes it into deep sleep without side effects. The sleep medication table on page 74 shows the many different options in each category. To see real improvement, most patients need to be on at least one medication or supplement from column 1 to increase deep sleep, so this is where I start. If needed, I'll then add a medication or supplement from column 2, a sedative that helps people fall asleep and stay asleep. If my patients are still having difficulty sleeping, or if their sleep is disturbed by nightmares, I'll add a treatment from column 3 to block the stress response. The good news is that some medications have dual action; for example, trazodone both acts as a sedative *and* slows brain activity into deep sleep.

Some of these medications have good research behind them, with studies showing that they increase deep sleep or are otherwise helpful for sleep in fibromyalgia. In those cases I have provided the reference. Others I have learned about through patient experience, what is known in medical research as anecdotal evidence. Many people prefer to avoid prescription medications when possible. I usually find that we do need to use at least one prescription to see significant improvement in sleep—most often one of the deep-sleep promoters—but I have had a few patients do really well with supplements alone.

Consult the table on page 74 with your HCP to find the right combination of medications for you.

FAQ: Is it safe to take multiple sleep medications together?

In general as long as you are *only* taking the medications listed on page 74, and *only* one from each column, there shouldn't be contraindications. Each column represents a different class of medicine that works on a different part of the brain. Problems can occur when you take multiple medications within the same class that are all acting on the same part of the brain. For example, you wouldn't want to take two sedatives like eszopiclone (Lunesta) and zolpidem (Ambien) together, as this could cause oversedation. It is also very important never to combine any sedative with alcohol or benzodiazepines, which can result in dangerous side effects such as excessive sleepiness, decreased breathing while sleeping, and even death. Work with your HCP to taper off any benzodiazepines before starting any new sleep medication.

Combining two sleep medications can also cause an additive effect, in which you may tolerate each on its own but when using them together may suffer from morning grogginess or other side effects. To reduce that risk I recommend starting only one medication or supplement at a time, beginning with a very low dose that slowly increases over several weeks. Once you are stable and tolerating it well, you can add a medication from another column, starting at a low dose and gradually working up. Your HCP will help determine the right dosage increase schedule for each medication.

How to Use the Sleep Medication Table Safely

The table on page 74 is to be used in collaboration with your HCP.

- All dosing refers to bedtime dosing.
- Talk with your HCP before you start any of the over-the-counter or herbal supplements listed.
- Never combine any sedatives with alcohol.

Medications and Supplements to Improve Sleep

Deep Sleep Promoters	Sedatives	Stress response blockers
Anticonvulsants	**"Z-drugs"**	**Muscle relaxants**
• gabapentin (Neurontin) 100–1,200 mg (Foldvary-Schaefer 2002) • pregabalin (Lyrica) 25–200 mg (Hindmarch 2005; Roth 2012) • topiramate (Topamax) 25–50 mg	• zolpidem (Ambien) 5–10 mg (Moldofsky 1996) • eszopiclone (Lunesta) 1–3 mg (Drewes 1991; Grönblad 1993) • zaleplon (Sonata) 5–10 mg	• cyclobenzaprine (Flexeril) 5–20 mg (Moldofsky 2011) • tizanidine (Zanaflex) 2–8 mg
GABA medications	**Sedating antidepressants**	**Alpha-blockers**
• baclofen (Lioresal) 5–20 mg (Huang 2009; Brown 2011) • tiagabine (Gabitril) 2–8 mg (Mathias 2001; Walsh Jan 2006, Apr 2006)	• trazodone (Desyrel) 25–200 mg (Mendelson 2005) • amitriptyline (Elavil) 10–30 mg • nortriptyline (Pamelor) 10–75 mg • doxepin (Sinequan) 1–6 mg • mirtazapine (Remeron) 7.5–45 mg (Schittecatte 2002; Yeephu 2013)	• clonidine (Catapres) 0.1–0.3 mg (Hunt 1986) • guanfacine (Tenex) 1–3 mg • doxazosin (Cardura) 1–8 mg • prazosin (Minipress) 1–6 mg
Supplements		**Low-dose antipsychotics**
• GABA 250–750 mg plus glycine 1,000 mg • magnesium 300–900 mg (Held 2002)	**THC derivatives** • dronabinol (Marinol) 2.5–10 mg • nabilone (Cesamet) 0.5–1 mg (Ware 2010) • medical marijuana	• ziprasidone (Geodon) 5–20 mg • quetiapine (Seroquel) 12.5–100 mg (Hidalgo 2007)
	Supplements • melatonin 1–10 mg • herbal sedatives: valerian root/hops (Dimpfel 2008)	

Medications to Increase Deep Sleep

The most important way to improve deep sleep in fibromyalgia is to take a medication or supplement that can slow down brain activity while you are sleeping. As you recall, in normal deep sleep brain waves are slow, but in fibromyalgia deep sleep is interrupted by fast "wakeful" brain waves. So using a medication to slow brain waves can force the brain into deep sleep and block some of those wakeful waves. Some work by increasing a chemical called GABA in the brain. Others slow down the electrical signals that brain cells send to each other. The most common side effects are grogginess and sedation.

Gamma-aminobutyric acid (GABA) is an amino acid the human nervous system uses to slow messages between nerve cells. Two medications that improve deep sleep by increasing GABA levels in the brain are baclofen and tiagabine. Baclofen is a muscle relaxant and antispasm medication. It is actually a distant cousin of Xyrem, the effective deep-sleep-inducing medication that has not been approved by the FDA for fibromyalgia. Baclofen has been shown to increase total deep-sleep time, and although not as strong as Xyrem, it can be a useful addition to your sleep regime, especially if you experience muscle cramps or spasms (Huang 2009; Brown 2011).

Tiagabine (Gabitril) also increases levels of GABA in the brain and slows brain activity while sleeping (Mathias 2001). In fact, it can nearly double the amount of time spent in deep sleep, and subjects given tiagabine have reported more restorative sleep and performed better on memory testing (Walsh Apr 2006). The major negative is that it comes with a risk of seizures, even in people without a previous history. For this reason it is usually my last choice in this group.

GABA can also be taken directly as a supplement; however, it is not well absorbed by the brain since its molecules are too big to easily permeate from the bloodstream. Thus it must be taken with glycine, another amino acid that does easily cross into the brain and carries the GABA along with it. Glycine also acts as an inhibitory neurotransmitter and helps slow down brain activity, so the combination of GABA and glycine can have an additional calming effect.

Magnesium supplementation can also increase GABA in the brain, but only through high doses. In one small study, magnesium supplementation increased the amount of time spent in deep sleep (Held 2002). It is also a good choice if you have any restless legs symptoms or nighttime muscle cramps, as it can reduce both.

FAQ: What is the best magnesium supplement?

Some forms of magnesium are not well absorbed by the intestines, magnesium oxide in particular. Magnesium citrate and glycinate are the most absorbable, and the usual dosage is 300–900 mg at bedtime. However, magnesium can act as a laxative—citrate more than glycinate—so if it is causing excessively loose stools, reduce the dosage to one that you tolerate. My favorite form is Natural Calm, a powder that when combined with warm water turns into highly absorbable form of magnesium citrate. I recommend one or two scoops at night, which can be a nice ritual before bedtime.

Anticonvulsants, which are used to prevent seizures, make up the other category of medications that slow brain activity. They work by slowing electrical impulses between nerve cells, which is also how they calm sleeping brain activity and support deep sleep. Pregabalin (Lyrica) and gabapentin (Neurontin) are anticonvulsants that have been shown to increase the time spent in deep sleep (Foldvary-Schaefer 2002; Hindmarch 2005; Roth 2012). These are among the most commonly prescribed medications for fibromyalgia pain, so if a patient is already taking one, I adjust to a higher dosage at bedtime. For example, if a patient on gabapentin 300 mg three times a day comes to see me, I might have them try 300 mg in the morning and 600 mg at bedtime. This tends to allow greater tolerance of the medications, which can cause grogginess or sleepiness when taken during the day. Topiramate (Topamax), another anticonvulsant that improves deep sleep, also reduces headache frequency and is a good choice for chronic headache or migraine sufferers.

Sedatives

The hallmark of fibromyalgia is poor sleep quality, but many patients also have insomnia—difficulty falling or staying asleep (not everyone does, though, so you may not need anything from this category). For this I recommend medications that are considered "sedative-hypnotic," a class of drugs used to induce and/or maintain sleep. Sometimes this can be as simple as taking melatonin, a hormone made naturally by your brain to induce sleep. It is a very safe treatment for insomnia with few side effects, especially at low dosages; a few patients have told me that higher doses (above 5 mg) increased their depression. The blood pressure medicines called beta-blockers (metoprolol, atenolol, labetolol, carvedilol, propranolol) block melatonin production, so patients on those medications should take at least 1–3 mg melatonin at bedtime (Stoschitzky 1999).

Herbal sedatives such as valerian root, chamomile, hops, passionflower, and rhodiola tend to be well tolerated. In one study, a combination of valerian root and hops helped subjects to fall asleep more quickly and induced more deep sleep than a placebo (Dimpfel 2008). Make sure to discuss any herbal supplements with your HCP before taking them. Although they are generally mild, like all medications they can cause side effects. I like a formula made by Thorne Research called Sedaplus, and I've also seen positive outcomes with a similar product from Pure Encapsulations called Best-Rest Formula.

For the most part, sedatives help you to fall asleep and stay asleep, but they don't do much to improve deep sleep, with a few exceptions. Trazodone is an antidepressant that is very sedating and has a long history helping people fall asleep; it also slightly increases deep sleep. Because of these dual effects, it is one of the more effective sedatives I have found for fibromyalgia (Mendelson 2005). Mirtazapine is another sedating antidepressant shown to increase deep sleep (Schittecatte 2002). It also reduces stress response activity in the brain, so is commonly used for PTSD. Mirtazapine has a twofold benefit for fibromyalgia since is both a sedative and a stress blocker. Tricyclic antidepressants such as amitriptyline, nortriptyline, and doxepin can work as sedatives and are a good choice for someone with peripheral neuropathy (nerve pain), which these medications can help reduce.

If a patient is on anything that increases serotonin levels, I tend to be cautious about introducing an antidepressant sedative, to avoid the risk of serotonin syndrome (see FAQ). Your HCP can help determine if any of the sedating antidepressants would be appropriate for you.

FAQ: What is serotonin syndrome?

Serotonin syndrome occurs when someone takes high doses of several medications that all act to increase serotonin levels in the brain. The most common culprits are antidepressants, migraine medications, and certain opiate-based pain medications, especially tramadol. Herbal supplements, including St. John's wort and 5-HTP, can also boost serotonin, as can the over-the-counter cough suppressant dextromethorphan. Symptoms of serotonin syndrome range from anxiety, shivering, and diarrhea to muscle rigidity, fever, and seizures. In severe cases, it can be fatal. Ask your pharmacist or your HCP about the risks associated with any new medications, especially if you are already on high doses of opiates, antidepressants, or tramadol, or take migraine medicine. If you suspect you might have serotonin syndrome after starting a new drug or increasing a dosage, seek emergency medical treatment.

The most commonly prescribed sedatives for insomnia are known as the "Z-drugs": zolpidem (Ambien), eszopiclone (Lunesta), and zaleplon (Sonata). Z-drugs are distant cousins of benzodiazepines (like the antianxiety medications clonazepam or lorazepam). They bind to the same brain receptors as benzodiazepines, but they do so in a very different way. This is an important distinction, because benzodiazepines have a negative impact on sleep (and some other side effects too; see FAQ), while Z-drugs have a neutral or even positive effect on sleep quality in fibromyalgia. For example, eszopiclone alleviates the fatigue caused by fibromyalgia and does not negatively affect deep sleep, and zolpidem improves daytime energy as well (Drewes 1991; Grönblad 1993; Moldofsky 1996). However, some HCPs do not feel comfortable prescribing the Z-drugs due to concerns about causing abnormal sleep behaviors or dependence, so they may be more willing to prescribe some of the other sedative options listed in column 2.

FAQ: I heard that using sleep medications like zolpidem (Ambien) can cause dementia. Is that true?

We don't know for sure, but it seems that some sedatives (including benzodiazepines and the Z-drugs) may increase the risk of developing dementia. Two studies looking at large populations of elderly patients found that those using benzodiazepines chronically had higher rates of dementia. One of these studies included the "benzodiazepine-like" Z-drugs, along with benzodiazepines. The other looked only at true benzodiazepines and did not examine Z-drugs. In both, the group on sedatives had significantly higher rates of dementia (Billioti de Gage 2012, 2014). However, anxiety and insomnia can be early signs of dementia, so it's not clear if the sedatives contributed to the development of dementia, or if people who were developing dementia had early symptoms that triggered a need for sedatives.

Overall these medications tend to be well tolerated, but they can occasionally have concerning side effects called "complex sleep-related behaviors." These abnormal reactions may include sleepwalking, sleep-eating, and, most alarming, sleep-driving. Patients describe waking up and finding candy wrappers all over their bed, or half the food in their fridge gone, with no memory of getting up at all. This is quite rare, but when it happens it tends to be dramatic and even dangerous. These behaviors generally occur within the first few days of therapy and are more frequent with zolpidem, so if you have a history of sleepwalking or abnormal sleep behaviors you should not take that drug. If anyone reports sleepwalking or sleep-eating while on zolpidem I have them stop treatment immediately.

That said, zolpidem is one of the medications that I most frequently prescribe for insomnia, for a few reasons: it is cheap and effective, and most people tolerate it just fine. Sedating antidepressants are often not an ideal option, because my patients are already on other medications that boost serotonin levels. Z-drugs, which don't affect serotonin, are a safer choice from the perspective of serotonin syndrome risk.

The other thing to know about zolpidem is that it's an amnestic, meaning it blocks memories. So people will take a dose and then read a chapter of a book or talk to their spouse and have no memory of it the next day. This can understandably be very disturbing to some patients, but is only a temporary effect of the medication. Eszopiclone does not have this amnestic effect, but it can cause a metallic aftertaste that bothers some people—one of my patients described waking up feeling like she had been "eating pennies" all night. Zolpidem, eszopiclone, and zaleplon can all cause several days of rebound insomnia if stopped suddenly, so you should work with your HCP to taper off if necessary.

You also should be aware that the Z-drugs stay in your system for around eight to ten hours, so you should only take them on nights when you have a full ten hours before you need to be up and active in the morning. In 2013 the FDA decreased the recommended dosage of zolpidem for women from 10 mg to 5 mg, after studies reported that 15 percent of women who took the 10 mg dosage still had enough medicine in their system to impair driving ability eight hours later (FDA 2013). (These results were not found in men, because they process the medication faster.) This occurred even more often with the long-acting form (Ambien CR), which I usually avoid altogether.

Another sedative that is not a Z-drug is now on the market in the United States, and it works in a very different way to induce sleep. Suvorexant (Belsomra) blocks the actions of orexin, one of the wakeful chemicals in the brain. By blocking orexin, it changes the brain from wake to sleep mode. So far, in my limited experience, it seems to work well and have few side effects, but as a newer medication it is very expensive.

Marijuana and medications derived from marijuana such as nabilone and dronabinol can help people fall asleep, and also show mild increases in amount of deep sleep (Feinberg 1975). Fibromyalgia subjects reported improved quality of sleep and feeling more rested in the morning after taking nabilone at bedtime (Ware 2010). You will learn about marijuana as medicine in chapter 21.

FAQ: If I take zolpidem (Ambien) every night, will I become addicted to it?

Taking zolpidem, or any of the Z-drugs, nightly will cause your brain to build up a tolerance to the point that suddenly stopping the medication might lead to several nights of difficulty sleeping. This is called dependence, and it is different than addiction. Dependence means that your body becomes used to a medicine and sudden cessation leads to symptoms of withdrawal. To avoid rebound insomnia, taper off the medication rather than stopping it abruptly. (Addiction, meanwhile, refers to abuse of medication—using it to get high. While it is possible to become addicted to the Z-drugs and misuse them, it is very rare.)

Medications That Block the Stress Response in the Brain

Some patients benefit from a medication to reduce the wakeful brain waves that interrupt deep sleep. Certain medications can reduce their occurrence by blocking the alarm signals being sent out by the hypothalamus, the part of the brain that controls the stress response. I find this especially helpful in patients who have nightmares from PTSD or who wake up with a start. Steve, my patient with PTSD, found huge sleep improvement when we added prazosin to block the stress response and reduce nightmares.

Tips on Choosing a Medication with Your HCP

- If you're on beta-blockers: melatonin
- If you have nightmares or PTSD: prazosin or doxazosin
- If you have bipolar depression: low-dose antipsychotics
- If restless legs are an issue: magnesium
- If you have chronic headaches or migraines: topiramate
- If you have peripheral neuropathy pain: tricyclic antidepressants

---

Medications that block the stress response are blood pressure medications called alpha-blockers, and antipsychotics. Muscle relaxants including tizanidine and cyclobenzaprine reduce it as well. Cyclobenzaprine is commonly used for fibromyalgia and has been shown to increase deep sleep and reduce fatigue (Moldofsky 2011).

Alpha-blocker medications (clonidine, guanfacine, prazosin, doxazosin) that are used to treat high blood pressure reduce the alarm signals in the brain. These medications can lower blood pressure, but most of my patients tolerate them in the low doses used for sleep. They can also cause orthostatic hypotension, a drop in blood pressure when moving from lying down to sitting or standing, resulting in feeling dizzy or lightheaded. I caution patients taking an alpha-blocker to get up slowly when lying down, and if they have a history of fainting or severe low blood pressure I avoid these medications.

Clonidine has the additional benefit of increasing growth hormone (Hunt 1986), and because of that it is often my first choice of the alpha-blockers. Growth hormone, important for repair of muscles, tends to be low in fibromyalgia. For anyone with PTSD-related nightmares I recommend prazosin or doxazosin, as they have been shown to reduce nightmares (Boehnlein 2007).

Some antipsychotics also act to block the stress response, especially quetiapine (Seroquel) and ziprasidone (Geodon), and have been shown to reduce fibromyalgia symptoms (Calandre 2012). Researchers saw improved sleep quality and reduced fatigue in patients taking quetiapine for sleep (Hidalgo 2007). I have found this type of medication most helpful for my patients with bipolar depression in addition to fibromyalgia.

I know that the many treatment choices described here might feel overwhelming, but just start with one and go from there. Maureen, the retired nurse, noticed a huge improvement in sleep once we added gabapentin at bedtime, and we didn't have to add any additional prescriptions. This information is probably the most important in the entire book, so spend as long as you need to working with your HCP to improve your sleep (I know, I'm a broken record). The process may take a little while, but without it the other treatments won't help as much. Be patient. I encourage you to reread this chapter and then make an appointment with your HCP to talk through your options.

To Do Yourself

- Reread this chapter and the last.
- Make an appointment with your HCP to discuss sleep treatment. Bring the HCP guide with you to that appointment.

- Bring a list of any of the sleep medications that you have tried before. Write down whether a medication was helpful for sleep and any side effects you can remember. This will speed up the process of finding effective treatments you will tolerate well.
- Talk with your HCP before starting any new supplements.

To Discuss with Your Health Care Provider

- Inquire if she is willing to review pages 249–273, the health care provider guide in the appendix, and then work with you to find a successful sleep treatment.
- Ask to start only one medication at a time. Begin with low doses and work up slowly.
- If she is unwilling to work with you to find a successful sleep medication combination, request a referral to a sleep specialist.

CHAPTER 10

Repair: Digestion

In the Rest chapters you learned important techniques to induce the relaxation response. Helping your body rest is fundamental to fibromyalgia treatment, and the more time you can spend doing it the better. Repairing the digestive dysfunction caused by a hyperactive stress response is the next step toward healing.

How the Stress Response Affects Digestion

Digestion is the process in which food is broken down into very small particles that can be absorbed and used by the body. It starts with chewing—mixing food with saliva in the mouth. The food is then swallowed into the stomach, where it mixes with gastric juice containing hydrochloric acid and pepsin, an enzyme that starts the breakdown of protein. Stomach acid serves a vital role in the absorption of many nutrients, including protein, B_{12}, iron, magnesium, calcium, zinc, copper, and vitamin C. From there, food moves into the small intestine, where it mixes with enzymes secreted by the pancreas. These pancreatic enzymes break it into particles small enough to be absorbed by the cells of the small intestine, where most of the nutrients are absorbed. The remainder is then passed into the large intestine, where water and some minerals are ingested into the body. Finally, waste is eliminated through the rectum.

Digestion is completely controlled by the rest-and-digest portion of the autopilot nervous system. The chronic fight-or-flight response in fibromyalgia results in impaired digestion because it reduces stomach secretions and impairs blood flow to the stomach and intestines. This results in inadequate stomach acid, which is essential for the breakdown of proteins and absorption of certain nutrients such as iron and B_{12}. The pancreas also does not produce enough enzymes, leading to inadequate breakdown of fats and carbohydrates. The fight-or-flight response also leads to increased permeability of the intestines, often called "leaky gut," which allows large undigested proteins and food particles to enter the bloodstream and cause inflammation.

Repairing Digestion in Fibromyalgia

I have all my patients start with at least one month of an intensive gut repair program before adding any supplements. It is pointless to take medicine that you are not going to be able to absorb! Focusing on gut repair first ensures that once you do start taking any additional supplements your body can actually use them.

Only once a leaky gut is repaired can we stem the tide of inflammation from food sensitivities. Strengthening digestion to ensure that food is broken down into its smallest particles and fixing leaky gut are essential first steps. After intensive gut repair we can then isolate any remaining sensitivities and make diet adjustments as needed.

My gut repair program improves digestion, restores healthy gut bacteria with probiotics, and heals the intestinal walls with glutamine supplements. Simple ways to improve digestion are to chew food well, eat slowly, take digestive enzymes with meals, and avoid acid-reducing medication. Mechanically breaking down food into as small pieces as possible makes it easier to digest. You can also boost the process by making sure you're relaxed during meals. Yes, this means not eating in the car, at your desk, or while distracted.

To boost digestive power, you can take enzyme supplements with meals. The most effective are those that contain stomach acid, usually in the form of betaine hydrochloric acid, along with pancreatic enzymes. Keep in mind that it is not safe to take acid-containing digestive supplements if you have stomach ulcers; it can make them worse. Both steroid medications and nonsteroidal anti-inflammatories (NSAIDs) increase the risk of developing stomach ulcers, so if you take either of those medications regularly it is best to avoid acid-containing digestive enzymes. Instead, take digestive enzymes without hydrochloric acid that contain only pancreatic enzymes.

Common Symptoms of Low Stomach Acid

- Feeling full after taking a few bites of food
- Indigestion
- Heartburn
- Nausea after taking supplements
- Weak, peeling, cracked fingernails
- Iron deficiency
- Undigested food in stool
- Bloating and belching after meals
- Chronic candida infections
- Bacterial overgrowth in small intestines

Many people end up on acid-reducing medications for symptoms of gastroesophageal reflux disease (GERD), which include nausea, heartburn, belching, bloating, and flatulence after meals. Unfortunately, acid-reducing medications have a negative effect on digestion: they impair absorption of certain vitamins and minerals, predispose to intestinal infections, and increase the risk of developing food sensitivities (Untersmayr 2008; Pali-Schöll 2010). I often recommend that patients stop or lower their dosage as part of strengthening digestion, but make sure to talk to your HCP first, as people with certain medical conditions, such as severe GERD or stomach ulcers, do need them.

Interestingly, the symptoms of low stomach acid often mimic those of excess stomach acid. Naturopathic doctors believe that the underlying cause of GERD is not an overproduction of acid, but actually an underproduction. The theory is that low stomach acid levels cause the sphincter muscle on top of the stomach to relax, allowing what little stomach acid there is to reflux and cause heartburn. A healthy, often higher amount of stomach acid can keep the lower esophageal sphincter muscle tight, preventing acid from reaching the esophagus.

Medications Prescribed to Lower Stomach Acid

omeprazole (Prilosec)

lansoprazole (Prevacid)

dexlansoprazole (Dexilant)

esomeprazole (Nexium)

pantoprazole (Protonix)

rabeprazole (Aciphex)

famotidine (Pepcid)

cimetidine (Tagamet)

ranitidine (Zantac)

FAQ: Can I take digestive enzymes with hydrochloric acid if I take acid-reducing medicine for gastroesophageal reflux disease (GERD)?

If you have mild to moderate symptoms of GERD it is worth talking to your HCP about stopping acid-reducing medications and trying digestive supplements. It seems counterintuitive, but I have found that many patients with mild to moderate GERD have fewer symptoms once they start digestive enzymes with hydrochloric acid. Remember, one theory is that GERD is caused by low stomach acid, not high. If you have been diagnosed with GERD, talk to your HCP before trying them out. For people with severe GERD or stomach ulcers it's not safe to take any supplements that contain hydrochloric acid. If you cannot tolerate acid-containing supplements I recommend one that contains only pancreatic enzymes and no hydrochloric acid, like Mega-Zyme by Enzymatic Therapy, which will also boost your digestive power.

Fixing a Leaky Gut

One of the biggest effects of a chronic stress response is a leaky gut, which is like a garden hose filled with thousands of holes. You even see it in lab rats subjected to prolonged stress, but not in rats whose adrenal glands have been removed so they cannot make stress hormones, indicating the connection between stress and intestinal permeability (Meddings 2000). Similarly, prolonged activation of the stress response in fibromyalgia leads to increased gut leakiness. Normally the gut only absorbs very small food molecules, which are familiar to the immune system and do not trigger an immune response. People with fibromyalgia on average allow nearly twice as many large particles through their small intestinal wall as control subjects (Goebel 2008). The immune system mistakenly recognizes them as foreign attackers, so they are more likely to bring about symptoms of inflammation such as fatigue and pain.

Reducing Leaky Gut

- Minimize use of NSAIDs.
- Take probiotics.
- Take L-glutamine 500 mg three times a day.

After optimizing digestion, the next step is to reduce gut leakiness and plug some of the larger holes in the hose. We first need to limit medications that worsen the problem. The biggest offenders are the nonsteroidal anti-inflammatories (NSAIDs), like ibuprofen or naproxen, which increase intestinal permeability within twelve hours of ingestion (Bjarnason 1995). Instead of NSAIDs, try turmeric and fish oil, which do not cause increased gut leakiness, or alternative prescription anti-inflammatories. You will learn more about these supplements and medications in chapter 14.

L-glutamine, an amino acid that is the primary fuel for the cells of the small intestine, has been shown to reduce gut leakiness (Quan 2004; Xu 2014; Rapin 2010). I start all my patients on two months of L-glutamine supplements. At that point, supplementation can be extended for people with significant digestive issues or multiple food sensitivities. During this time of intensive gut repair I also prescribe probiotics, healthy bacteria that enhance intestinal barrier function and reduce gut leakiness (Mennigen 2009; Ukena 2007). Probiotics also help with irritable bowel syndrome, and this dual action is why they are one of the core supplements that I recommend taking on an ongoing basis.

Calming Irritable Bowel Syndrome

About 70 percent of patients with fibromyalgia also have irritable bowel syndrome (IBS) (Veale 1991), so the final step in repairing digestion is to reduce its symptoms: abdominal pain, bloating, constipation, diarrhea, and nausea. Alternating bouts of constipation and diarrhea are common.

IBS reflects a digestive system that is operating in fits and starts, like a car with a transmission problem. Efforts to induce a relaxation response and more time spent in rest-and-digest mode will help reduce its symptoms.

I also recommend a daily probiotic supplement to restore a healthy balance of bacteria in the intestine. One study found that four weeks of probiotics (*Bifidobacterium lactis, Lactobacillus rhamnosus,* and *Streptococcus thermophilus*) lessened IBS symptoms in 68 percent of patients (Yoon 2014). To keep up a diverse balance of intestinal bacteria I recommend changing brands every few months to ones with different species. Avoiding foods that cause food sensitivities can also help reduce IBS. In chapter 14, you will learn how to eliminate the most likely offenders.

Trusted Probiotic Brands

VSL#3
Enzymatic Therapy
Jarrow
PB 8

There may also be a link between small intestine bacterial overgrowth (SIBO) and IBS. Normally, bacteria in the human digestive tract live mostly in the large intestine. The small intestine should contain only a small population. When the bacteria in the small intestine grow out of control, it causes SIBO and leads to impairment of digestion and absorption of nutrients. The bacteria produce methane and hydrogen gas in abundance, causing bloating, abdominal pain, excessive gas, and belching. SIBO may contribute to irritable bowel syndrome, with reports of small intestine bacterial overgrowth in almost 40 percent of IBS sufferers (Pyleris 2012). It is diagnosed with a breath test that measures how much methane or hydrogen gas you exhale after ingesting a specific type of sugar that only bacteria can digest. The test is usually done at gastroenterology clinics; many naturopaths also offer it. SIBO is treated with a course of antibiotics, usually rifaximin for ten to fourteen days, along with a low-carbohydrate diet to starve the bacteria of nutrition (Quigley 2006).

Finally, it's time to get rid of food efficiently by avoiding constipation. As a doctor, I talk about poop. A lot. And it's astonishing to me that most people do not think they are constipated, even when they have obvious clues. If I ask, "Do you have regular bowel movements?" most patients answer, "Yes." To someone who is used to pooping only once a week, this *is* "regular." So I have learned to ask more specific questions, like "What does your poop look like?" Healthy poop should look like a banana or a snake, and be smooth and soft. If it looks like rabbit pellets or pebbles, you are constipated! I also ask exactly how often they have bowel movements. If you go three days or more between, you are constipated!

The longer food sits in your GI tract, the more toxic waste products are produced that can cross through a leaky gut. Avoiding constipation may require laxatives like magnesium or polyethylene glycol (MiraLAX), along with increased fiber and water. Everyone taking opiates for pain needs a daily laxative—possibly a strong one like senna or bisacodyl—as these medications are *extremely* constipating. Opiates slow down the waves moving waste through the bowels. Many patients on opiates don't even realize they are constipated until they get an abdominal X-ray for some other reason and the report comes back as "bowels filled with stool."

FAQ: Is it dangerous to take laxatives daily?

Taking certain types of laxatives regularly can cause your bowels to get lazy and not work as effectively on their own. However, mild laxatives like magnesium or polyethylene glycol (MiraLAX) can be safely taken every day.

To Do Yourself

- Take digestive enzymes with meals.
- Minimize use of NSAIDs.
- Start one to two months of intensive gut repair with L-glutamine and probiotics.
- Avoid constipation.
- Read about SIBO diagnosis and treatment at www .siboinfo.com.
- If you want to learn more about IBS, read *A New IBS Solution: Bacteria—the Missing Link in Treating Irritable Bowel Syndrome* by Mark Pimental, MD.

To Discuss with Your Health Care Provider

- If you have GERD, ask your HCP before starting any digestive enzymes that contain hydrochloric acid.
- If you think you might have SIBO, talk with a naturopath or holistic provider about getting tested.

CHAPTER 11

Repair: Therapeutic Movement

While you are working on repairing digestion as discussed in the last chapter, it is the perfect time to add in techniques to boost blood flow to and repair your tissues. You can do this with gentle exercise and bodywork focused on the fascia.

More than eighty studies have shown that exercise reduces pain and fatigue in fibromyalgia (Jones May 2009). The challenge is that when you hurt all over and are exhausted, the last thing on earth you want to do is exercise. Trust me, I know! When I was diagnosed, everything I read said that regular exercise was important, but it just made me feel worse. I often felt like I had strained a muscle, and my muscles felt even more achy and tight afterward. I also frequently injured myself while exercising; tight fascia makes us more prone to do so. It wasn't until I learned how to really gently warm up my muscles and fascia that I was finally able to tolerate exercise and benefit from it.

So let's throw the word "exercise" out of our vocabulary and think of it as "therapeutic movement." Our muscles *do* need to move to be healthy, but in such a way that it is therapeutic, not harmful. When used as medicine, exercise (sorry, therapeutic movement!) can repair the ability of your muscles and brain to make energy. It also brings more blood flow to tissues to heal painful areas of the fascia. Combined with manual therapy directed at the fascia, it is a particularly powerful method of repairing tissue function and reducing pain.

How Exercise Helps in Fibromyalgia

- Releases endorphins, the body's natural painkillers.
- Increases blood flow to the brain and improves memory and cognition.
- Reduces tension in fascia.
- Promotes deep sleep.
- Triggers growth hormone release.
- Produces more mitochondria to make energy.
- Increases joint fluid production and reduces arthritis pain.

Warming up tight muscles and fascia is the key to getting benefit from exercise. Warm, relaxed muscles are much less likely to get hurt than cold, tight ones. Many people think that stretching first will do the trick, but that is not a true warm-up; nor is walking slowly on a treadmill or doing a low setting on an exercise bike. A good warm-up is non-weight-bearing, and involves slowly moving key joints and muscles through a gentle range of motion. This both increases blood flow to the joints and gently stretches the tight fascia around the joints and muscles, boosting their lubrication and your ability to tolerate exercise without injury or pain. As physical therapists like to say, "Motion is lotion."

This gentle stretching of the fascia prepares your muscles to move. Excess fascial tension caused by a hyperactive stress response means it takes longer to get the juices flowing and the tissues loose and warm. Working with a sports medicine expert, I developed a warm-up program specific for fibromyalgia. I have fine-tuned it over the years and use it personally and share it with all my patients. It has made all the difference for me in being able to benefit from exercise. After Maureen, the retired nurse, started doing this warm-up, she was able to tolerate walking on a treadmill. In fact, she found that exercise began to reduce her pain levels—exactly the result we want!

The warm-up starts with deep breathing to activate the relaxation response and encourage the tight fascia to soften. Next is gentle movement of the toes, then the ankles, the knee and hip joints, and finally the shoulders.

How to Warm Up

The first step is to get warm—literally. Raise your body temperature by sitting in a nicely heated room, taking a hot shower or bath, or lying under a blanket. If you are going to a gym, wear several layers that you can remove once you start moving. Warmth is essential to an effective warm-up, because muscles are already looser when your temperature is slightly elevated.

Go through the warm-up described and illustrated below. Spend as long as you like in each stage, but don't focus too much on any one body part, and make sure to frequently alternate your motions so as to not cause strain on one particular area. If a movement doesn't feel right to you, slow it down, skip it, or modify it in a way that feels better. A video is available at www.fibromanual.com so you can see the moves, and potential modifications, in action.

1. **Lie down.** On a yoga mat or carpet, lie on your back with hands at your sides, feet shoulder width apart, and legs flat on the ground.

2. **Breathe.** Take slow deep breaths. Think about allowing your pelvic muscles to relax, and your body to soften and feel heavy against the floor.

3. **Toe curl.** Slowly curl and extend your toes a few times on both feet.

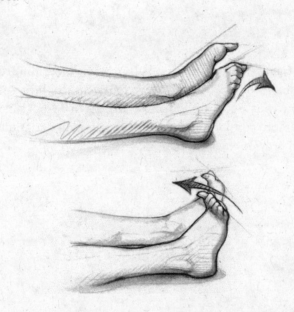

4. **Ankle flex and circle.** Bend your knees toward your chest and place your hands on your knees. Point and flex your feet slowly a few times, continually but gently moving your ankles through their full range of up-and-down motion. Rest a few seconds, then gently circle your ankles through their full range of motion. You can do both ankles at once or one at a time. (See the illustration on the next page.)

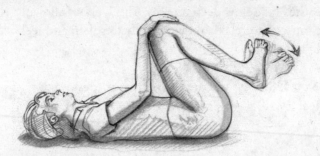

5. **Foot shake.** In the same position with knees toward your chest, shake your feet up and down for twenty to thirty seconds, allowing your ankles to flop and your legs to be loose like jelly. If it is more comfortable, place your hands under your lower back to provide extra support.

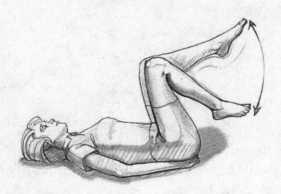

6. **Basic position.** Put your feet back on the floor, with your knees bent. This is the basic position. (See the illustration on the next page.)

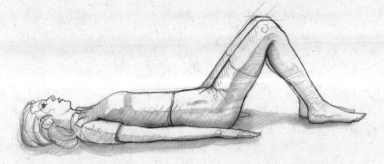

7. **Knee to chest.** From the basic position, bring one knee toward your chest and then return your leg to the basic position. Bring the other leg toward your chest, and then back to the basic position. Alternate legs and do this four or five times on each side. If it is more comfortable, place your hands under your lower back to provide extra support.

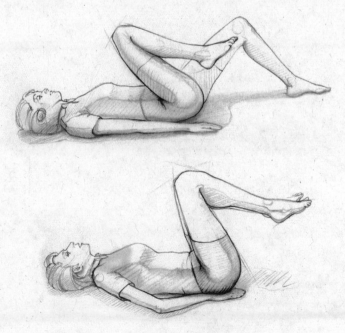

Supporting the lower back.

8. **Chest-extend-chest-replace.** From the basic position, bring one leg toward your chest, then straighten that leg so that it is a few inches above the ground. Bend your leg back toward your chest, then place it on the floor. The pattern is chest-extend-chest-replace. Do this on both legs, four or five times each. If it is more comfortable, place your hands under your lower back to provide extra support.

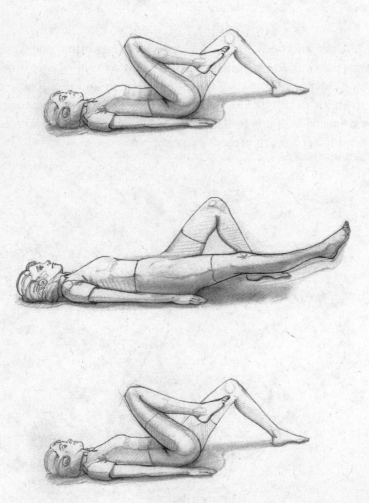

9. **Chest-extend-lift-replace.** From the basic position, bring one leg toward your chest, straighten it so that it is a few inches above the ground, lift it toward the ceiling in the air, then bend it and return to the basic position. The pattern is chest-extend-lift-replace. Do this three or four times with each leg. If it is more comfortable, place your hands under your lower back to provide extra support.

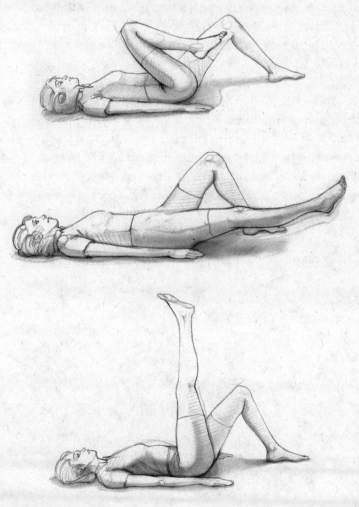

10. **One leg lifted, ankle circles.** From the basic position, lift one leg straight up with your hands behind your thigh for support. The other leg can either remain flat on the floor or bent at the knee with your foot on the ground if that is more comfortable. Allow the back of your thigh to stretch for twenty to thirty seconds, then point and flex your foot a few times. Make very slow circles with your foot, putting your ankle through its range of motion. Allow your foot to stay in each position for a few seconds as it moves around the circle. This provides a nice stretch of all the muscles and fascia in the foot and ankle. Switch legs and repeat.

11. **Air bicycle.** Still lying on your back, bring your knees to your chest so that your knees and feet are both above your abdomen. Place your hands underneath your lower back to stabilize your pelvis, and then make gentle circling motions with your legs, as if you were riding a bicycle. Try to have your feet over your chest, not your pelvis, to reduce strain on your back. Do this for ten seconds, rest, then repeat for another ten seconds.

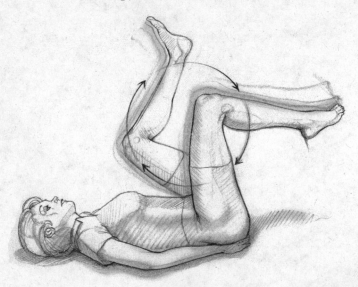

12. **Shoulder roll.** Stand up with feet shoulder width apart. With arms hanging loosely at your sides, do some gentle shoulder rolls forward and backward.

You are finished with the basic warm-up. It should take less than ten minutes to do the whole thing. Now you can do a few key standing stretches and then you'll be ready to exercise. The stretches that I find most helpful are described below; you might have other areas that you like to work on before jumping in. However, leave the majority of stretching until after you complete your routine, when it benefits your muscles the most. And don't spend more than one or two minutes stretching after the warm-up, or you will cool down before you even start exercising.

The calf stretch. Face a wall, standing two to three feet away from it. Lean your forearms on the wall, keeping your head, neck, and spine in a straight line.

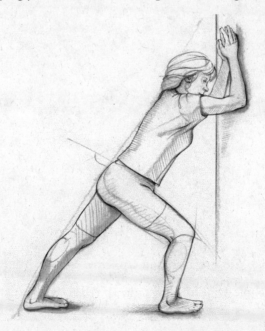

Now bend one knee and bring that knee forward toward the wall. Keep your other leg straight with the heel down. Do this stretch for twenty to thirty seconds, then switch to the other calf. This stretch is really important, because it can reduce some of the pressure of the plantar fascia in the foot, which tends to be very tight and prone to injury.

The thigh/shin stretch. Bending forward at the waist, straighten one leg and put the heel of that foot on the ground. Bend the other leg slightly at the knee, and support your arms on the thigh of the bent leg. It is important to keep your back as straight as possible during this stretch. Do this for about ten seconds on each leg.

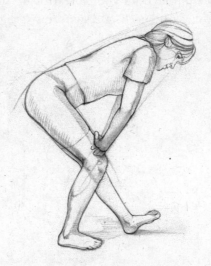

Now That You Are Warmed Up, How Should You Exercise?

Many people with fibromyalgia are so fatigued that they are only able to tolerate very small amounts of exercise. For some of my patients I have them start with the warm-up routine alone, at least twice a week. Then, as tolerated, I ask them to add one minute of gentle walking, and then some stretching. Over time, they slowly add another minute, and then another.

Often people with fibromyalgia (myself included) start an exercise program by trying to do the customary twenty to thirty minutes recommended for weight loss and cardiovascular health, but suffer so much in the days following that they give up completely. Our goal is not to lose weight or get in shape—this is exercise as *medicine*.

A patient once told me that she had started doing warm-water therapy pool exercise, but always felt wiped out for three days afterward, so she stopped going. When I asked her how long she customarily stayed in the pool, her answer was, "Ninety minutes, because it felt so good." That is a guaranteed recipe for disaster! My mantra here is "start low and go slow." Avoid group exercise at first, since peer pressure can cause you to push beyond your limits.

My personal exercise regimen started with the warm-up, then just a few minutes on the elliptical machine, and then stretching. Over the years, I have worked my way up to twenty- to twenty-five-minute elliptical sessions. Whenever I fall off the exercise wagon for a time, I start again with very short sessions and build up slowly. Even with small amounts of gentle exercise, it is best done only every two to three days, to give your body adequate recovery and repair time. As you read in previous chapters, inadequate deep sleep and lower growth hormone means that it will take you a little longer to recover. It is crucial to give yourself that time before going at it again.

I have also learned to increase the length of exercise sessions gradually, not push myself too hard, and to listen to my body when it says *Stop!* I recommend a very low-impact exercise such as walking or using an elliptical machine or recumbent exercise bike. Exercising in warm-water therapy pools—at a temperature of 88–92°F, roughly the temperature of a luke-warm bath—has been shown to be very well tolerated in fibromyalgia (Gowans 2007). It may also provide additional benefits, as the warmth can help reduce muscle pain, spasm, and stiffness.

Strength training is generally not well tolerated unless it is very low intensity; in fact, it's the only exercise out of the eighty studies I mentioned that did *not* show benefit for fibromyalgia. If you still want to add strength training, I recommend it only after you have built up your tolerance for aerobic exercise, and keep weights and repetitions very low. The water resistance of pool-based therapy is one way to gently build muscle and strength.

Exercising the Right Way for Fibromyalgia

- Warm up every time.
- Choose low-impact activities.
- Start low and go slow.
- Allow at least a forty-eight-hour recovery period between sessions.

Balance and Exercise

When using exercise as medicine, it's important to be aware that about half of people with fibromyalgia report balance problems, ranging from mild to severe. In particular, we have a hard time maintaining balance when asked to do a secondary cognitive task—like subtracting sevens backward from 100 while walking—but tend to score normally in seated tests (Jones Feb 2009). We don't know exactly why, but it may be a result of poor signaling from the muscles and joints to the brain; the brain gets confused about where the body is in space. It is also possible that a brain that is distracted by constant pain signals has less capacity to devote to activities like maintaining balance.

Some of my patients are more impacted than others. If you have poor balance and frequent falls, choose exercises that are low to the ground, like the recumbent bike, and hold the handrails on the treadmill or elliptical machine. Activities like yoga that involve balance may be helpful, but be sure you do standing postures by a wall or other support. One of my patients found that regular use of the Wii Balance Board, which has games and yoga postures, improved her balance and was fun to use. A few studies have found that regular use of the Balance Board improves balance and strength (Nitz 2009; Clark 2010).

Low Blood Pressure and Exercise

Many people with fibromyalgia have low blood pressure that can drop even further after they stand up, due to the effects of the chronic fight-or-flight response on blood vessels (Furlan 2005). Severe drops in blood pressure may lead to palpitations, dizziness, and fainting. To avoid this, get up slowly from any seated or lying position, especially while exercising. Try eating small amounts of protein every two hours.

The most effective way I have found to treat this is with saltwater, because salt naturally increases your blood pressure (this is why people with high blood pressure are told to lower their salt intake). I recommend just a pinch of sea salt in each glass of water—not so much that it tastes salty. Think of it as a sports drink without the sugar. A year after my diagnosis, I was drinking twenty glasses of water a day and still feeling dehydrated and often on the verge of fainting. After my naturopath recommended saltwater, those symptoms went away. I find it actually quenches my thirst and I have to urinate *less* frequently throughout the day, because salt helps keep water in your bloodstream and brings blood pressure levels up into the normal range. If you have high blood pressure in addition to fibromyalgia, discuss it with your doctor before starting to drink saltwater.

Warm-Up Summary

I can never remember the whole regimen in order, so I usually bring a list in my pocket to the gym. Here is a warm-up summary that you can photocopy and take with you, or post by your exercise machine at home. There is also a video available at www.fibromanual.com that guides you through the warm-up.

The Warm-Up

1. Lie down	7. Knee to chest
2. Breathe	8. Chest-extend-chest-replace
3. Toe curl	9. Chest-extend-lift-replace
4. Ankle flex and circle	10. One leg lifted, ankle circles
5. Foot shake	11. Air bicycle
6. Basic position	12. Shoulder roll

To Do Yourself

- Practice the warm-up routine with the video available at www.fibromanual.com.

- Remember to start low and go slow as you work on therapeutic movement.
- If you have low blood pressure or dizziness, add one-quarter teaspoon sea salt to sixteen ounces of water and drink at least twice daily.

To Discuss with Your Health Care Provider

- Ask if it is safe to start a new exercise program given your current physical condition.
- If you have high blood pressure, ask before adding any salt to your water.

CHAPTER 12

Repair: Unsticking the Fascia

My muscles feel bunched up in knots.
—NEARLY EVERY PERSON WITH FIBROMYALGIA

First we improved your body's ability to break down food and absorb nutrition. Then we stimulated blood flow to the tissues through exercise. The final stage of Repair is to restore the structural integrity of the myofascial system (muscles and fascia) by loosening tight, painful adhesions. In fibromyalgia the continual fight-or-flight alarm means that both the muscles and the fascia are tense and ready for battle. The fascia is the connective tissue "armor" of the body, tightening immediately in response to signals from the many nerves running throughout it. This provides strength in emergency situations and can be lifesaving in the short term. But the sustained tightness of the fascia that we see in fibromyalgia results in tissue inflammation and painful adhesions and knots called trigger points.

Patients with fibromyalgia have some distinctive muscular abnormalities, not in the muscles themselves, but in the connective tissue that encases them, the fascia. Biopsies show an unusually high number of immune cells and excess collagen.

There is growing data that pain from the fascia generates fibro-myalgia muscle pain, and this has been my personal, clinical, and research experience (Liptan 2010). Interestingly, this theory is not actually new at all. Over a hundred years ago a physician named William Gowers theorized that "inflamma-tion of white fibrous tissue" was the source of fibromyalgia pain (at that time called fibrositis or chronic rheumatism) (Gowers 1904). His theory gained support when muscle biopsies of these patients indeed showed abnormalities in connective tissue (Stockman 1904). But research shifted from the muscles toward the brain, until recently, when myofascial release (a manual therapy directed at the fascia) was shown to promote lasting pain reduction for fibromyalgia patients.

Two European studies found that after twenty sessions of myofascial release, which focuses on gently stretching the fascia that surrounds every muscle, fibromyalgia subjects reported significant pain reduction. What is really great, though, is that they also showed long-lasting pain relief, with reduced levels after one month and six months after their last session (Castro-Sánchez 2011, Sep 2011). I led a pilot study that confirmed these results and found that myofascial release therapy (MFR) relieved pain much better than standard Swedish massage (Lip-tan 2013).

MFR is by the far the most effective treatment I have found to unstick the fascia and reduce fibromyalgia pain. When I stumbled across it after being diagnosed, I saw a huge improve-ment in my pain levels, particularly in my back, neck, and jaw. I also noted changes in the way my body felt: my tissues finally started to relax. For days after treatment, I slept deeper and woke up feeling less tight. Looking back on it from a medical perspective, the therapy was reducing the fight-or-flight ner-vous system influence so my tissues could unlock. Indeed, studies have shown that gentle stretching of the fascia does ac-tivate the relaxation response (Cottingham 1988). Now if I do even a few minutes of self–myofascial release techniques using a ball or foam roller, it quickly helps me relax and reduces tightness. I found that the best way to talk to my brain is through my fascia!

Ways to Unstick the Fascia

- Myofascial release
- Structural Integration (Rolfing)
- Self–myofascial stretching
- Yin yoga
- Trigger point injections or dry needling
- Microcurrent therapy
- Gentle exercise

What Exactly Is the Fascia?

Before we delve into fascia treatment, let's take a step back and learn more about this fascinating body structure that has until recently been ignored by the mainstream scientific community. If you were to ask your doctor about the fascia, she might not be able to tell you much, because "medical books barely mention fascia and anatomical displays remove it" (Grimm 2007).

On my first day of gross anatomy class in medical school, after cutting into our cadaver I was shocked to see that every muscle was covered in a tough and beautiful iridescent white coating. You probably have seen an outer layer of fascia in the translucent covering you peel away from a chicken breast. The fascia is the connective tissue that surrounds and supports every muscle in the body, along with forming the tendons that insert into bone. It encloses every bundle of muscle fibers and even each individual muscle cell. Each muscle is made up of thousands of long springs—the muscle cells—bound together into a tight bunch by multiple layers of connective tissue wrapping. When scientists take a muscle biopsy, they can chemically dissolve the actual muscle cells and examine the fascia, an intricate honeycomb of connective tissue. This network of tissue is highly sensitive to pain and actually has more nerve endings than the muscle cells themselves (Stecco 2007; Kellgren 1938; Bonica 1990).

The fascia is made up of a thick gel called the extracellular matrix and cells called fibroblasts. These cells secrete the components of the "goo" that surrounds them, and produce tough fibers of collagen and stretchy fibers of elastin. Think of the fibroblast as a spider weaving a web of extracellular matrix. It is the gel-like properties of the fascia that cause it to become solidified with ongoing tightness. But with gentle sustained pressure, the gel can also return to a softer, more elastic state as well. And that is exactly what myofascial release does.

Reducing Tension in the Fascia

The fascia is a very dense gel, like a solid block of taffy, that can be molded and stretched only with slow and sustained pressure. The fibroblasts inside the gel respond positively to slow stretching by secreting chemicals that accelerate the healing process in the tissue around them. Several manual therapies provide just the right amount and type of pressure needed to stimulate the fibroblasts and loosen those tight and dense areas. The primary one I recommend is myofascial release (MFR), a combination of sustained manual traction and prolonged gentle stretching. Studies show that the gentle sustained pressure of myofascial release speeds up tissue healing and reduces inflammation (Cao 2015). Standard massage techniques do *not* stimulate fibroblasts or address fascial tightness, which may be why many people with fibromyalgia don't find much benefit from standard massage therapy.

If you gently bend your head to the side right now, as if trying to rest your ear on your shoulder, you will feel a pulling or stretching sensation on the opposite side of your neck, from shoulder to jaw. What you are feeling is not actually stretching of the muscle—there is no one muscle that runs from your shoulder to your ear—but stretching of the fascia surrounding all the muscles between those two points. If a myofascial release practitioner were to put one hand on your shoulder and one near your jaw and leave them there for several minutes, this gentle stretch would help ease any tightness in that area.

I recommend that patients try at least two or three MFR sessions to determine if it will help them. It may temporarily cause increased muscle soreness, similar to what you feel after intense exercise. But after a day or two the muscle pain should be much better than it was prior to the session. If you find it helpful, I recommend going once or twice a week for about eight weeks, similar to a typical schedule for physical therapy. After that it can be done as needed for pain flares. Most therapists will also teach you techniques using balls or other tools that you can do at home to extend the benefit of each treatment.

FAQ: Is myofascial release the same as deep tissue massage?

Unfortunately, "myofascial release" has become widely and inappropriately used as a generic term for deep tissue massage, and many practitioners conflate the two. Some athletic trainers also teach foam roller techniques that they call myofascial release. Deep tissue massage or foam rolling is *not* helpful in fibromyalgia. When I refer to myofascial release I mean the gentle prolonged stretching of the fascia of the John F. Barnes' Myofascial Release Approach. See the chapter resources for information on how to find a trained therapist.

There are several ways to stretch your own fascia and get many of the same benefits as myofascial release therapy. Ideally this would be done in combination with receiving some MFR from a professional, but if that is not an option, you will still see improvement from doing these stretches on your own. Additional resources for at-home techniques are listed at the end of the chapter. Learning these self-care tricks may be the most important step you take to manage your pain, and are a huge emphasis in my clinic's treatment program.

You can treat yourself by placing a small, soft ball under any tight and painful area. Allow yourself to sink onto the ball for a few minutes to provide the right amount of sustained pressure to simulate myofascial release.

I also really recommend the CranioCradle, a small, soft foam cushion that you place under your neck or upper or lower back for a nice fascial stretch. It's also an effective way to induce a relaxation response, as discussed on page 51. Doing this for three minutes a day is a simple way to reduce pain and promote relaxation.

Other Treatments for the Fascia

Structural Integration, or Rolfing, is a manual therapy that approaches fascial treatment a little differently. A form of hands-on manipulation developed more than fifty years ago, Rolfing focuses on the fascia around the joints, with treatment emphasizing correcting posture and joint alignment in a series of ten to twelve sessions. One of my patients benefited so much that she was inspired to become a practitioner and now treats fibromyalgia patients herself!

A similar therapy is osteopathic manipulative treatment (OMT), a combination of gentle stretching and pressure on the muscles and joints. Since OMT is performed by osteopathic physicians (DOs instead of MDs), it is often covered by insurance.

Yin yoga is a slow, gentle form of yoga that includes supported stretching using props such as pillows and bolsters to settle into a comfortable position for several minutes, allowing the fascia to melt and soften. Check out yin yoga classes or videos to learn and practice the poses.

Gentle aerobic exercise and stretching can also reduce tension in the fascia, but it is important to carefully warm up muscles prior to exercise, as you learned in the previous chapter.

Microcurrent Therapy

Very low levels of electricity—a microcurrent—also have beneficial effects on the fascia. The level used for therapy is below what we can feel, and is much less than that used in a TENS (transcutaneous electrical nerve stimulation) unit, a common pain treatment. It causes the muscle and fascia to vibrate, unsticking and softening tight areas, and may also stimulate repair mechanisms in tissue. In rats, it was found to increase ATP (the energy currency of cells) by 500 percent. It also increases protein production and movement, both of which are important for tissue repair (Cheng 1982). In one study, eight weeks of treatments brought neck myofascial pain levels down from an average of seven to two (McMakin 1998). Another reported similar results for low back myofascial pain caused by trigger points (McMakin 2004).

Microcurrent is also thought to reduce inflammation in the tissue. Research in fibromyalgia patients found that the treatment reduced pain levels and lowered inflammatory markers in the blood (McMakin 2005). A few myofascial release therapists use microcurrent treatment either before or after a treatment, and the combination of the two seems particularly effective for pain reduction in some patients.

Trigger Points

Myofascial trigger points are "hot spots" in the fascia that irritate nearby muscle cells, causing them to contract. Trigger points often develop after injury, mechanical stress, or repetitive microtrauma—all conditions under which the fascia becomes "sticky." This combination of contracted muscle cells and sticky fascia creates a taut, painful lump or band. When the fascia is already contracted and irritable, it is very easy to develop these hot spots, and trigger points are quite common in fibromyalgia. One study found an average of twelve in subjects with fibromyalgia, with healthy controls having one or none (Alonso-Blanco 2011).

Focusing on treating those trigger points can reduce local muscle pain. The most effective treatments involve physically disrupting the tissue by stretching, massage, or insertion of a needle into the muscle. Think about a snag in a sweater, and the bunching or knot of fibers that it causes. The only way to unravel the knot is to pull the fibers away from each other and slide them back in place. A trigger point is essentially a snag in the fiber of the fascia, and these sticky fibers need to be physically released or broken up to allow the muscle to relax.

Trigger point injections—inserting needles with a numbing

medicine—that break up these tissue knots have been shown to be helpful in fibromyalgia (Staud 2014). One study found reduced muscle pain compared to placebo injections that were done near, but not into, trigger points (Affaitati 2011). Another showed reduced pain and increased range of motion in fibromyalgia patients after trigger point injection (Hong 1996).

Some physical therapists also offer dry needling, the use of needles alone to break up the trigger point. It has also been shown to be effective, but the addition of numbing medicines reduces the intensity and duration of post-injection soreness (Hong 1994).

Focused, intense finger pressure and some other massage techniques can also undo a contraction knot. A technique called "spray and stretch" puts a numbing medication on the skin and then performs intense stretching to break up a trigger point. The Thera Cane is a cane-shaped tool that allows you to place deep pressure on your own trigger points in the upper back and neck and is a low-cost option.

Whatever method you choose, softening the tight and knotted areas of fascia can dramatically reduce muscle pain.

To Do Yourself

- To learn more about the John F. Barnes' Myofascial Release Approach or find a therapist in your area, visit www.myofascialrelease.com or www.mfrtherapists.com.
- To learn more about Rolfing, or to find a therapist in your area, visit www.rolf.org.
- To find an osteopathic physician (DO) who performs OMT, go to www.osteopathic.org.
- Learn how to do self–myofascial release with *Myofascial Stretching: A Guide to Self-Treatment* by Jill Stedronsky and Brenda Pardy.

- Visit www.craniocradle.com for helpful instructional videos on self–myofascial stretching techniques.
- Thera Cane is a cane-shaped tool that allows you to place deep pressure massage on trigger points in the upper back and neck: www.theracane.com.
- To learn more about treating your own trigger points, check out *Healing Through Trigger Point Therapy: A Guide to Fibromyalgia, Myofascial Pain and Dysfunction* by Devin J. Starlanyl and John Sharkey, and *The Trigger Point Therapy Workbook: Your Self-Treatment Guide for Pain Relief* by Clair Davies and Amber Davies.
- To learn about microcurrent therapy and find a practitioner, visit www.frequencyspecific.com.

To Discuss with Your Health Care Provider

- Ask for a prescription or order for myofascial release therapy. It is most often done by massage and physical therapists. If you have a prescription, insurance may cover it.
- Ask for help identifying any trigger points, and if you have some, request trigger point injections. If your HCP does not perform them, request referral to a provider who does, usually pain specialists, physiatrists (physical medicine and rehabilitation specialists), and sports medicine specialists.

CHAPTER 13

Rebalance: Energy Production

Once your body has absorbed nutrients from food, it must transform that fuel into energy for your cells. In fibromyalgia, energy production is inefficient and out of balance, which is especially deleterious to those tissues that require the most energy—the muscles and brain (McClave 2001). Together, they use almost half of all the body's energy. Not surprisingly, then, the symptoms of fibromyalgia manifest primarily in these two areas. When the brain cells aren't able to make enough energy to keep up with the body's demand, we experience fatigue. When the muscle cells aren't able to make enough, it results in muscle pain and weakness. Fibromyalgia muscles have lower than normal amounts of the energy-carrying chemical ATP, and people with fibromyalgia have a reduced tolerance for exercise, with muscles that easily fatigue (Park 1998; Gerdle 2013; Bachasson 2013). Improving the ability to produce energy from nutrients is a key factor in restoring balance and reducing fatigue and muscle pain.

An Energy Imbalance

A single cell in the human body may contain as many as one thousand mitochondria, which are like the engine of a car. The food you eat is the gas, and how far you can drive on a tank is related to how efficiently the car's engine makes energy from fuel—the gas mileage. Chemicals released during the stress response are major regulators of fuel metabolism, and they push the mitochondria to make fuel quickly—but not efficiently (Elenkov 2000).

The brain is the largest consumer of energy in the body, but in proportion to other organs it has fewer mitochondria. So the mitochondria in our brain cells work very hard, making the brain especially sensitive to mitochondrial dysfunction. Mental fog and fatigue reflect a brain that is not getting adequate fuel.

The muscle cells also suffer, because the fight-or-flight nerves tell them to quickly produce as much energy as they can from stored fuel in order to fend off a threat. Due to constant muscle tension, they also burn through fuel, like continually idling a car with very bad mileage—you go through a lot of gas! This perpetual misuse of muscle energy means that you blow through nutrients faster than they can be replaced, and build up painful waste products. It's why we've already focused so heavily on reducing fascial and muscle tension in order to stop idling the engine.

Improving Mitochondrial Function

To restore balance to energy production we need to use high-quality fuel in the form of nutrition that will improve the mileage of your cell's engines. Gradually incorporating aerobic exercise trains muscles to become more efficient at generating energy, and increases the number of mitochondria in each muscle cell. It's like adding extra engines to your car! Exercise also helps remove old and unhealthy mitochondria (Ding 2013). Increasing evidence suggests that it can also make more mitochondria in tissues beyond the muscles, including the liver, brain, and kidneys (Little 2011).

To improve your mileage, we first need to cut out things that harm mitochondria, and then add nutrients to boost their energy production. Mitochondria need glucose and oxygen to make energy, so anything that limits their ability to access either of those reduces their capacity. For example, if there are not enough red blood cells to carry oxygen to other cells, as in anemia, it hampers mitochondrial energy production. Smoking cigarettes also interferes with oxygen delivery, and in illnesses like diabetes or pre-diabetes the body struggles to get glucose from the bloodstream into cells, which makes it harder for mitochondria to make energy. So quitting smoking and getting your blood sugar under control if necessary will enhance your energy production.

You can also boost the ability of your mitochondria to make energy by giving them easily digestible fuel. Mitochondria function best with stable blood sugar levels, so don't skip meals, and eat frequent high-protein snacks. Mitchondria love healthy fats, so eat foods rich in omega-3 fatty acids like egg yolks, cold-water fish like salmon, and grass-fed beef. Cook with and eat high-quality oils like coconut and olive oils. See page 125 for ten mitochondrial "superfoods." Mitochondria also really like a form of sugar called D-ribose. Supplementation (generally 5 gm two to three times a day) has been shown to increase energy and reduce pain (Teitelbaum 2006). I have found D-ribose to be especially helpful for patients who experience extreme fatigue and muscle weakness after exercise.

We can also increase efficiency by adding specialized nutrients (carnitine, CoQ10, and alpha-lipoic acid) that allow the mitochondria to make more energy from that same amount of fuel. It like going from a car that gets ten miles a gallon to one that gets twenty (Parikh 2009).

Ten Superfoods for Mitochondria

Almonds (raw, not roasted)
Avocados
Blueberries
Broccoli
Grass-fed beef/buffalo
Green tea
Pomegranates
Salmon (wild, not farm-raised)
Seaweed
Spinach (organic)

Things That Harm Mitochondria

Anemia (low red blood cells)
Smoking tobacco
Low vitamin D levels
Toxins/pesticides
Poor diet
Diabetes/insulin resistance

Carnitine is an amino acid that acts like a key to open the door to transport fatty acids into the mitochondria so they can be oxidized ("burned") to produce energy. The most readily absorbed form is acetyl-L-carnitine. Carnitine in the diet comes from meat, so it is especially important for vegetarians to add this supplement. Ten weeks of acetyl-L-carnitine reduced overall fibromyalgia symptoms more than a placebo pill (Rossini 2007). Alpha-lipoic acid is a powerful antioxidant that increases the ability to convert fuel to energy in mitochondria, and studies on lab rats show that in combination with carnitine it improves muscle function (Sundaram 2006).

Coenzyme Q10 (CoQ10) is like a rechargeable battery that moves energy around as it is produced in the mitochondria, and supplements have been shown to reduce pain and fatigue in fibromyalgia patients (Cordero 2013). Some prescription medications for high cholesterol called statins deplete CoQ10 levels in the body, causing muscle pain and cramps (Ghirlanda 1993). If you take any statin medications it is essential to supplement with CoQ10 to limit that side effect. The usual recommended dose is 100–300 mg daily, but you should double this if you are on a statin. Note that it may decrease the effectiveness of blood-thinning medications such as warfarin (Coumadin) or clopidogrel (Plavix), so they should be taken together *only* under the careful supervision of your health care provider.

FAQ: What type of CoQ10 should I take?

CoQ10 comes in two forms: ubiquinol, the active antioxidant form, and ubiquinone, the oxidized form, which the body converts to the active form. Most supplements contain both. Theoretically, those containing only ubiquinol may have more of the active form and so may be more effective, but the jury is still out. In the meantime, you can take either as long as you remember that it is a fat-soluble vitamin—that is, it is not soluble in water—so it is important to take it with meals that contain fat to enable absorption.

Mitochondria also need B vitamins and magnesium. B vitamins need to be altered by the body to work correctly, so taking preactivated forms allows the body to use them more readily. You can find preactivated B vitamins, magnesium, and the right amounts of acetyl-L-carnitine, alpha-lipoic acid, and CoQ10 in a product called RevitalAge Nerve, by Pure Encapsulations. It's as close as I have found to an all-in-one supplement for mitochondrial support in fibromyalgia, but if you are on a statin you will still need extra CoQ10.

Start taking these supplements after completing the gut repair program discussed in chapter 10, so that you can absorb and utilize them most effectively. Keep in mind that you may not need to take these supplements forever. Often three to six months gives your system a reboot, and as long as you eat well and exercise you'll continue with more efficient energy production even once you stop.

Recommended Dosages of Mitochondria Support Nutrients

Acetyl-L-carnitine 1,000 mg daily
Alpha-lipoic acid 400–600 mg daily
CoQ10 100–300 mg daily

Vitamin D for Mitochondria

Vitamin D is produced in the skin by exposure to sunlight, and we also get some when we eat eggs, fatty fish such as salmon and mackerel, and fortified dairy products. It is best known for its role in calcium absorption and bone health, but it is also critical for muscle repair and mitochondrial function (Eyles 2005). People with low levels of vitamin D often have poor mitochondrial function, causing diffuse musculoskeletal pain and weakness (Sinha 2013; Bouillon 2013). The good news is that mitochondrial energy production can recover with supplementation.

FAQ: Should I take prescription or over-the-counter vitamin D?

I find the over-the-counter form (cholecalciferol, or D_3) to be more effective—and in fact it has been shown in two studies to be better than the prescription (ergocalciferol, or D_2) at raising serum vitamin D levels (Heaney 2011; Binkley 2011). Some doctors prescribe high-dose weekly pills for patients with very low blood levels, but that version is synthetic and not as easily absorbed or used by the body.

In fibromyalgia, it is particularly important to take a vitamin D supplement, since it is so important in muscle and mitochondrial function. I usually recommend between 1,000 and 5,000 IU daily, depending on blood levels (see text box below). The in-range level is 60–80 ng/ml, and anything higher than 150 ng/ml may have negative side effects. Since vitamin D is fat-soluble, it is best absorbed in the intestine along with fats, so I recommend the oil-based gel capsules.

Recommended Daily Vitamin D_3 Based on Blood Levels

Vitamin D level less than 30 ng/ml → 5,000 IU daily and repeat blood levels in three months

Vitamin D level 30–60 ng/ml → 2,000 IU daily

Vitamin D level greater than 60 ng/ml → 1,000 IU daily

Nutrition

To boost the ability of your cells to make energy, you need to give your body the highest-quality, most nutritious food you can. You probably already have some ideas about how to make your diet healthier: increase fruits and vegetables, and eat as much healthy protein and organic food as you can. Also, eating high-protein snacks every two to three hours provides fuel throughout the day. Many people with fibromyalgia do well with a Paleo-type diet, emphasizing meat, vegetables, and healthy fats and avoiding most grains and dairy. As you will learn in the next chapter, grains and dairy are inflammatory foods that may cause symptoms to flare. If you minimize processed foods, it's also easier to avoid food additives like MSG that can trigger pain.

The mitochondria, the energy producers of our cells, are especially sensitive to pesticides and other toxins we ingest, and unfortunately one recent study showed that two-thirds of produce in grocery stores had pesticide residue (EWG 2015). Certain foods hang on to chemicals more than others, so those are the ones to make sure to eat only organic. Of course, organic produce is more expensive, so if cost is a barrier, prioritize those foods that tend to be the most contaminated.

"Dirty Dozen" Fruits and Vegetables

Make sure to buy organic!

Apples	Sweet bell peppers
Strawberries	Nectarines
Grapes	Cucumbers
Celery	Cherry tomatoes
Peaches	Snap peas
Spinach	Potatoes

Source: www.ewg.org.

I always ask new patients what they ate for breakfast that day, and the answer is very revealing. About half the time people answer, "Nothing," or "A cup of coffee." I am about to tell you something you already know: eat breakfast every day! It really is the most important meal of the day, and when you skip it you start out with an energy deficit.

Most of us know the importance of a nutritious breakfast, but some mornings that's just too much to accomplish. It can be hard to eat healthy when you are in pain and too fatigued to go grocery shopping or cook a meal; it's much easier to grab quick processed foods. In medical school I was so ill that for a time all I could manage to eat were protein bars and take-out. Many of these dietary changes are things you already know you should be doing—actually doing them is the hard part, and I don't want to downplay that reality.

My patients have found various creative solutions, including ordering groceries online or buying prepared veggies and salads from the deli section at health food stores. Hard-boil a dozen eggs on Sundays for a quick energy-bump snack throughout the week. Adding a high-quality protein powder to a smoothie, or mixing it with rice or nut milk, is another easy way to boost your protein intake. I recommend MediClear by Thorne Research, a rice-and-pea-protein-based dietary supplement.

Starting with a few simple changes, like making sure to eat some protein at every meal, will make the next change a little easier. And don't feel that you suddenly have to eat nothing but salad and grilled fish. Remember, your diet does not have to be perfect; just add in higher-quality foods where you can, and you'll feel the results.

Easy Breakfast Ideas

Apple with nut butter

Rice cake with nut butter

Hard-boiled egg

Leftovers from dinner

Protein powder in a smoothie

Oatmeal with walnuts and raisins

Oatmeal with peanut butter

One thing that motivates me is the thought that the food I eat actually becomes part of my body. Your atoms, the very small particles that make up your tissues, come from the food you eat, the water you drink, and the air you breathe. I really don't want to incorporate that Pop-Tart into my body!

To Do Yourself

- Eat breakfast.
- Increase protein and healthy fats.
- Don't skip meals.
- Supplement your mitochondria with CoQ10, alpha-lipoic acid, and acetyl-L-carnitine.
- Quit smoking.

To Discuss with Your Health Care Provider

- Check vitamin D levels. Request vitamin D over-the-counter replacement, not the prescription form, which has been shown to be less effective.
- If you're on blood thinners, talk to your HCP before adding CoQ10.

CHAPTER 14

Rebalance: Inflammation

Inflammation, which is an activation of the immune response, is necessary for healing and tissue repair. But it must be kept in check, so the body has both anti-inflammatory and pro-inflammatory chemicals. In fibromyalgia this balance is lost and skews toward systemic inflammation, resulting in flulike feelings of achiness and fatigue that anybody with the disease knows well. Restoring a healthy equilibrium is key to reducing pain and fatigue.

The excess inflammation in fibromyalgia comes from several different pathways that all start with the chronic activation of the stress response. First, as we learned in chapter 12, the fascia is in a constant state of inflammation. Second, deep-sleep deprivation causes elevated levels of inflammatory chemicals in the body; this has been demonstrated in healthy volunteers who are deprived of deep sleep (Haack 2007; Lentz 1999).

You have already reduced the inflammatory load on your body with the healing actions in Rest and Repair. Getting more deep sleep will cut down on inflammatory chemicals in your body, as will efforts to lessen the tightness of the fascia, along with strengthening digestion and repairing a leaky gut.

However, if you have worked through all the Rest and Repair steps but are still having symptoms, there may be an underlying issue that needs to be addressed. Symptoms of excess inflammation include joint pain, flulike aching, rashes, skin irritation, sinus congestion, headaches, and irritable bowel. Hidden infections, such as chronic sinusitis or dental infections, can be potent triggers, as can foods that provoke an immune response. Here we'll discuss how to identify food sensitivities and infections, and how to use anti-inflammatory supplements and medications.

Sources of Inflammation in Fibromyalgia

- Lack of deep sleep
- Tension in the fascia
- Food sensitivities
- Chronic low-grade infections

What Is Inflammation, Anyway?

Anytime the body's immune system is activated it is called inflammation. The immune system mobilizes its chemical messengers to address a threat, causing various symptoms, most commonly muscle achiness and fatigue. If you have ever had the flu, the achiness you felt was due to your body's rapid release of a huge amount of inflammatory chemicals called cytokines and immune cells to fight off the virus. Several studies have found levels of inflammatory cytokines in fibromyalgia patients that were as high as those in the blood of someone with the flu (Bazzichi 2007; Wang 2008). Some cytokines tend to be elevated and some are lower than normal in fibromyalgia (in fact, this abnormal pattern of cytokines in the blood is one potential diagnostic tool) (Sturgill 2014). In addition, white blood cells from fibromyalgia patients don't respond normally when exposed to certain irritating substances in a lab. The cause of this is currently unknown, but it is most likely due to effects of the stress response interfering with immune function. The researchers who discovered this have developed what they market as "the first objective diagnostic test" for fibromyalgia, the FM/a (Behm 2012). This test, however, is based on only one study, so the results must be replicated before it becomes an accepted tool in medical practice.

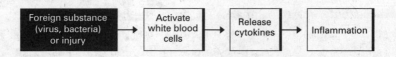

Pathway to inflammation.

FAQ: If there is inflammation, why does my doctor tell me that my markers are normal?

The usual blood tests for inflammation are indeed normal in fibromyalgia. Doctors generally look for blood markers called the ESR (also called "sed rate") and CRP (C-reactive protein). In fibromyalgia, the ESR and CRP are generally within range, which has led to the mistaken conclusion that there is no inflammation present. More specialized testing to look at cytokines shows clear evidence of inflammation, but this testing is currently only performed in research studies.

Finding Food Sensitivities

Food sensitivities are one of the biggest sources of inflammation in fibromyalgia and where we can make a huge impact on symptoms. A study of forty patients found that every single one tested positive for multiple food sensitivities. Half of the subjects maintained their usual diet and lifestyle (the control group), and the other made dietary changes to avoid allergens (the treatment group). At three and six months, the treatment group felt substantially better, with less pain and fatigue (Deuster 1998).

Remember that large, poorly digested food particles are more likely to trigger an immune response. The steps you took to strengthen digestion and repair a leaky gut will reduce your sensitivity, but unfortunately we can't completely restore everything to normal due to the ongoing stress response; there may still be some large particles sneaking through and causing an immune reaction. Symptoms aren't usually felt right away—the response (body aches, fatigue, headache, and flulike feelings) happens over several hours or days. If you're still feeling these types of symptoms even after improving digestion and leaky gut, we need to find out which foods you are sensitive to so you can limit your exposure. What I tell my patients is that most people with fibromyalgia do have some sensitivities, but not all to the same foods. We'll figure out your specific needs by starting with the most common triggers: gluten, dairy, and sugar. I was amazed to find that when I stopped eating gluten the constant ache in my knees went away. Now I can always tell when I have accidentally eaten something with it, because my knee pain flares up . . . my knees are my gluten sensors!

FAQ: Isn't the whole gluten-free thing just another fad diet?

Gluten—a protein found in wheat, barley, and rye, and any products made with those grains—has been in the news a lot recently. Many doctors are skeptical that so many people could suddenly have developed a gluten sensitivity. While I can't speak to society at large, in fibromyalgia I find that many, but not all, patients feel less pain and fatigue once they stop eating gluten. A leaky gut leaves us prone to developing immune responses to foods, and gluten is a highly irritating substance to the immune system. Someone without a leaky gut or other factors triggering their immune system may tolerate gluten just fine, but with fibromyalgia patients I always recommend they avoid it for two months to judge for themselves.

Methods to Find Food Sensitivities

- IgG antibody test to food
- White blood cell reaction test
- Elimination/challenge diet

First, let's clarify the difference between food allergies and food sensitivities. Food allergies are fast immune reactions (minutes to hours) that are triggered by contact with food particles with IgE antibodies. The result is usually hives, swelling of the mouth, or breathing problems called anaphylaxis. Allergies are discovered by skinprick tests in which small amounts of the suspected substance are injected under the skin and the response of redness or swelling is measured. They can also be tested by measuring IgE antibodies in the blood. In contrast, food sensitivities are slower, causing a reaction over hours to days, and are triggered by food particles coming into contact with certain white blood cells or a different type of antibodies called IgG.

While the food allergy IgE blood tests are well accepted in Western medicine, the concept of food sensitivities is controversial. Testing and treatment for food sensitivities is generally done by alternative providers like acupuncturists, naturopaths, and chiropractors. Complicating matters further, there is no perfect diagnostic tool. The immune response is so complex and intricate that it makes finding sensitivities a little tricky. There are three ways that we can try to detect them, but each only gives part of the picture. The first is an elimination/challenge diet, which is considered the gold standard, meaning the most reliable and effective. It means cutting out all suspect foods (dairy, gluten, corn, soy, and eggs) for at least six weeks and then reintroducing them one at a time and observing your response. The biggest drawback is that it is hard to do. It is also limited in that it only looks at entire food groups, so it does not detect sensitivities to more specific foods like types of fruits, vegetables, or meats, nor food additives, colorings, preservatives, or spices.

The next test measures IgG antibodies in the blood to different foods, preservatives, and additives. IgG testing also reveals only part of the puzzle, because not all food sensitivities involve antibodies—many reactions are triggered directly from interaction with the white blood cells. The test that offers the most complete data is one that measures the reaction of white blood cells when exposed to different substances. Since white blood cells produce antibodies, this method goes to the heart of the issue to discover *both* antibody-related sensitivities and direct white blood cell reactions. I recommend the ELISA/ACT (Enzyme-Linked Immunosorbent Assay/Advanced Cell Test) as the most reliable and useful. I personally noticed a significant reduction in flulike achiness after eliminating foods that it identified.

FAQ: I've heard that nightshade vegetables are bad to eat if you have fibromyalgia. Is this true?

This is a myth that has been around for decades. In fact, nightshades like eggplant, peppers, potatoes, and tomatoes are no more likely to cause an immune response than any other food. I have certainly had patients who have found they were sensitive to one or all of these vegetables, either through an elimination diet or through sensitivity testing, but it is not a common sensitivity.

Here is the approach I recommend for my patients. First, try a modified elimination diet by avoiding the trifecta of the most common problem foods: gluten, dairy, and sugar. Linda, whom you met earlier, noticed a huge reduction in pain with a switch to eating Paleo (high protein, no dairy or grains, low carbs and sugar). Completely avoid all high-sugar foods, dairy products, and the grains wheat, barley, and rye, which contain gluten. It is important to read labels, as many packaged foods contain gluten or dairy ingredients. It takes about six weeks for your body to completely clear out old IgG antibodies, so you need to stick with it for at least that long (ideally eight weeks) before slowly adding back those food groups one at a time. If they *are* a problem, you will notice improved pain levels while off them and an exacerbation of symptoms when you add them back. Keep in mind that you might feel worse before better, so give it the full eight weeks before judging. If these avoidance trials are not informative but I still suspect food sensitivities, then I will order one of the blood tests, either IgG or ELISA/ACT.

If sensitivities are confirmed, I recommend completely avoiding those foods for six months before trying to reintroduce them.

With a break from that food the immune system can often reset and produce a lower or even no response when you try them again. Other sensitivities may not go away and you will need to continue avoiding those triggers. MSG and artificial sweeteners such as aspartame are very common catalysts for immune responses (not to mention being toxic to the brain) and are known to flare up fibromyalgia pain, so I recommend that everyone with fibromyalgia avoid them completely (Smith 2001). These are not the type of food sensitivities that will improve with some time away. You will learn more about the brain toxicity of MSG and aspartame and healthier alternatives in chapter 19.

FAQ: If I am sensitive to gluten, does that mean I have celiac disease?

Not all people who are sensitive to gluten have celiac disease. Celiac disease is a fairly rare condition in which the body's immune reaction to gluten causes injury to the wall of the small intestine. It is diagnosed by testing for specific antibodies to gluten or by a small bowel biopsy that shows damage to the small intestine, which can cause problems with absorption of nutrients. If I see a patient with very low levels of iron or B_{12} I always check for celiac.

Gluten sensitivity is much more common than celiac disease. It means that you experience discomfort after eating gluten, but do not have an immune reaction that damages the small intestine. It remains controversial in the medical community, but researchers are now describing a non-celiac gluten sensitivity, manifesting with abdominal pain, rash or eczema, fatigue, diarrhea, hand or foot numbness, and joint pain (Sapone 2012).

Supplements That Reduce Inflammation

Omega-3 fatty acids (usually in the form of fish oil or flaxseed oil) and turmeric are effective options for reducing inflammation. Fish oil has been shown to relieve symptoms in inflammatory diseases such as rheumatoid arthritis, asthma, and Crohn's disease (Simopoulos 2002). Multiple studies have shown that omega-3 supplementation results in reduced joint pain and less need for anti-inflammatory drugs in rheumatoid arthritis (Kremer 1995; Ruggiero 2009). Fish oil also increases endocannabinoids—natural anti-inflammatories similar to chemicals found in marijuana—which may be another reason it eases pain (Berger 2002).

Dietary sources of omega-3 are mostly in oils from fatty fish: anchovy, sardine, and mackerel. Because fatty fish can be contaminated with mercury or lead, make sure that the supplement you choose has been purified to remove heavy metals. I recommend 2,000–3,000 mg per day. Krill oil, which comes from small shrimplike creatures, has similar benefits. At 300 mg per day it can reduce arthritis pain and inflammation (Deutsch 2007). Flaxseed and borage oils are good plant sources of omega-3s.

FAQ: How can I stop having disgusting fish burps after taking fish oil?

Make sure to take fish oil with a meal, and keep your capsules in the fridge or freezer. The colder temperature keeps the oil encapsulated until after it leaves the stomach. Try different brands, as I've found that some people may tolerate one variety better than another.

Another anti-inflammatory supplement is turmeric, which has been used in India for medicinal purposes for hundreds of years. Turmeric is a plant related to ginger whose roots are dried and ground into a spicy orange powder. Its active ingredient is curcumin, which is also what makes it orange. Curcumin has similar anti-inflammatory effects to NSAIDs (nonsteroidal anti-inflammatory drugs), leading some to call it the "herbal ibuprofen" (Deodhar 1980). In fact, curcumin may be more effective at reducing pain and swelling in joints than NSAIDs for rheumatoid arthritis (Chandran 2012). In an eight-month study of one hundred osteoarthritis patients, supplementation with curcumin decreased arthritis pain and reduced inflammation (Belcaro 2010).

Curcumin is generally not well absorbed from the GI tract, so oral doses must be high to see an effect. In newer supplements the curcumin is bound to phosphatidylcholine, which is more easily absorbed, letting it piggyback a ride into the bloodstream. Meriva is a curcumin-phosphatidylcholine made by Thorne Research that I have found very effective. Usual dosage is 1,500–2,000 mg daily, divided, taken with meals to avoid nausea. Start low and slowly work up to full dose. It can be taken every day or just as needed for pain. The huge advantage of curcumin over NSAIDs is that it has fewer side effects such as ulcers and does not worsen leaky gut. However, just like NSAIDs, it has some blood-thinning effects, so you should avoid it if you are also taking prescription blood thinners such as warfarin. If you are unsure whether it is safe for you to take curcumin, make sure to ask your HCP before starting supplementation.

Medications to Reduce Inflammation

There are a few prescription medications I recommend to reduce inflammation in fibromyalgia, especially if you also have joint or back pain from arthritis. Because they worsen leaky gut I generally don't recommend oral NSAIDs, but topical application can be quite effective for arthritic joint pain. (See chapter 19 to learn more about using NSAIDs externally for pain relief.) An oral NSAID called celexocib (Celebrex) works a little differently and therefore causes fewer leaky gut issues. It is still not ideal to take every day, but as a just-as-needed medication it is a much better choice than common NSAIDs like ibuprofen or naproxen. I find it especially helpful for patients who have significant pain from arthritis too.

I also sometimes prescribe hydroxychloroquine (Plaquenil), which is used to treat autoimmune disorders such as rheumatoid arthritis, lupus, and Sjögren's syndrome. In these conditions, the immune system attacks the body itself, causing inflammation, which hydroxychloroquine blocks. Although fibromyalgia is not an autoimmune disease, some patients do have mild autoimmune-type inflammation, which can be seen in a positive antinuclear antibody (ANA) test. High ANA levels are seen in lupus, but if the results show only a slightly elevated antibody load, it is usually considered "normal" and disregarded. In my opinion, *any* positive ANA is still an indicator of excess inflammation, and patients with both fibromyalgia and slightly positive ANA tests often benefit from prescription anti-inflammatories. It takes about six weeks on hydroxychloroquine see any effect, and about six months for its full effect, so plan to give it at least a six-month trial. This medication does not cause leaky gut, but in rare cases it can lead to eye damage, so if you take it you need a yearly exam with an ophthalmologist. Any eye problems are reversible if caught early and the medication is stopped.

Colchicine is another anti-inflammatory that does not cause leaky gut. Egyptian medical texts from 1500 B.C. describe the use of its plant source, the autumn crocus (*Colchicum autumnale*), for treatment of joint pain. These days it is most commonly used to treat gout, a form of arthritis. Very low daily doses can be helpful for patients who have persistent elevated markers of inflammation. A low dose is key, because at higher levels it can be toxic to the liver or kidneys.

Both colchicine and hydroxychloroquine have some potentially serious side effects, so I only consider them when all other anti-inflammatory treatments have failed. They are generally prescribed by rheumatologists (who are experts in treating gout and lupus), not by primary care providers. So if you are interested in trying one of them, ask for a referral to a rheumatologist.

Finding and Treating Chronic Low-Grade Infections

The lack of deep sleep and the chronic stress response in fibromyalgia both reduce your ability fight off infections, and many patients' energy levels are dragged down by chronic subclinical infections. These smolder below the level of full-blown illness, but still aggravate the immune system and cause inflammation. The tonsils, sinuses, gums, teeth, intestinal tract, and vagina are the most common locations of subclinical infections. I have had several fibromyalgia patients whose symptoms improved after removal of chronic abscessed teeth or treatment for other protracted low-grade oral infections. If you suspect you may have an oral infection, I suggest visiting a dentist or oral surgeon for assessment. Newer imaging techniques such as conebeam CT scans provide much better images of periodontal bones and can find hidden or deep infections that aren't detected by X-rays (Tyndall 2008).

Other common hidden infections include yeast overgrowth causing chronic sinusitis or vaginitis. The human body is host to hundreds of different types of bacteria and fungi. The most common fungus, a yeast called *Candida albicans,* lives in every human body in warm, moist places like the sinuses and the vagina. Normally a delicate balance exists between yeast and bacteria in the mucous membranes, so that neither causes illness, but if this balance is disturbed it can lead to an overgrowth of fungus. Yeast overgrowth in the mucous membranes can trigger a body-wide inflammatory response. In people with fibromyalgia, *Candida albicans* was the second most likely culprit to elicit an immune response on the ELISA/ACT test (Deuster 1998).

Most Common Hidden Chronic Infections in Fibromyalgia

- Vaginitis
- Sinusitis
- Dental infections

Frequent antibiotic use kills the bacteria that usually compete with yeast for food, and can lead to excessive growth of yeast, as can taking steroids. The yeast that lives in our body, just like the yeasts used to bake bread, really likes sugar. So a high-sugar, carbohydrate-rich diet, combined with antibiotics or steroid medications, is a setup for yeast overgrowth. Common symptoms are chronic sinusitis and repeated or persistent vaginal yeast infections. Acute sinusitis often happens after you get a cold due to a bacterial infection, but once it becomes chronic, yeast is usually to blame. And indeed, chronic sinusitis patients have high levels of yeast in their sinuses, causing habitual inflammation (Taylor 2002; Ponikau 1999). Of course, most people with chronic sinusitis get treated with antibiotics, which just makes things worse. Yeast overgrowth can be detected by checking blood levels of antibodies to *Candida albicans*. Everyone will have some, because candida lives on and in all of us, but a high antibody load points to overgrowth.

To treat yeast overgrowth, reduce sugar and carbohydrates in your diet. Probiotics, which contain healthy bacteria like those found in yogurt, can also help reduce yeast levels. For severe cases, a course of antifungal medications may be needed as well.

To treat chronic sinusitis, in addition to these steps I recommend daily nasal irrigation with saline water to help rinse debris from your nasal cavity. Some people do this with a neti pot, a small pitcher that can be filled with saltwater and gently tipped into your nostril. It is important to use boiled or bottled water rather than tap water to avoid any bacterial contamination. The technique can be a bit tricky to master; it is often simpler to use a nasal saline spray. I like a brand called Simply Saline that has no preservatives.

That yeast overgrowth can cause chronic health issues is not accepted by most Western medical practitioners, so if you suspect that it may be a problem for you, I highly suggest seeking out a naturopath or holistic MD to help with diagnosis and treatment.

To Do Yourself

- Do an eight-week trial diet that avoids the trifecta of the most common inflammatory foods: gluten, dairy, and sugar. The Mayo Clinic (www.mayoclinic.org) has good information about eating gluten-free. More recipes and resources for a non-grain, non-dairy Paleo-type diet can be found at www.paleoleap.com, www.nomnompaleo .com, and www.thepaleodiet.com.
- Supplement with fish oil and turmeric (curcumin) to reduce inflammation.
- Read about yeast overgrowth in *The Yeast Connection Handbook* by Dr. William Crook.
- Take probiotics to balance out yeast and add more healthy

bacteria. Good probiotic brands include VSL#3, Enzymatic Therapy, Jarrow, and PB 8.
- If you suffer from chronic sinus infections, read *Sinus Survival* by Dr. Robert Ivker.

To Discuss with Your Health Care Provider

- If you take NSAIDs regularly, ask about changing to celexocib to reduce the risk of gut leakiness.
- If you are on blood-thinning medications, discuss before starting a turmeric (curcumin) supplement.
- Ask about food sensitivity testing. Genova Diagnostics, US BioTek, and the Great Plains Laboratory all offer IgG testing for food sensitivities. ELISA/ACT is for white blood cell reactivity testing (www.elisaact.com).
- Request a referral to a rheumatologist if you're interested in trying colchicine or hydroxychloroquine, especially if you have significant joint pain or persistent elevated ANA, ESR, or other inflammatory markers.
- See a naturopath if you're concerned you may have yeast overgrowth.
- See a dentist to check for oral infections.

CHAPTER 15

Rebalance: Adrenal Hormones

The hyperactive stress response in fibromyalgia can cause hormonal imbalances in the adrenal or thyroid glands. Issues with the adrenal and thyroid hormones can be major players in persistent fatigue for some, but not all, patients. As you recall from chapter 13, the chronic stress response in fibromyalgia results in mitochondria, the cells' energy producers, that don't function efficiently. And if the mitochondria in the thyroid and adrenal cells are not working well, you will get a poor hormone response from those cells.

The changes you have already made in the Repair section to boost mitochondrial function will improve your hormone response. High levels of inflammation also disturb hormonal equilibrium, so reducing inflammation, as you learned how to do in the previous chapter, will also help. For many patients, the Rest and Repair steps are enough to rebalance their hormones. But people with more complicated hormonal dysfunction may need further support. In particular, I see more severe imbalances in patients who also have chronic fatigue syndrome or hypothyroidism, or who take long-term high-dose opiates.

Given all the interactions between the various hormonal systems, balancing them is a delicate dance. Think of the three major hormone systems—adrenal, thyroid, and sex—as levels of a house, one atop the other. Adrenals form the foundation, and if they are off balance, the thyroid and sex hormones will be erratic as well. We cannot restore balance to the thyroid or sex hormones without first stabilizing the adrenals. Thus the most important place to start is by addressing adrenal dysfunction.

Adrenals Are the Glands of the Stress Response

The adrenals are two grape-size glands that sit on top of each kidney. Their primary function is to produce the stress hormones cortisol and adrenaline. They also make aldosterone, a hormone that signals the kidneys to retain salt to regulate fluid balance, and small amounts of the sex hormones testosterone, estrogen, and progesterone.

Cortisol levels fluctuate throughout the day, helping to regulate the sleep/wake cycle. Normally levels are higher in the morning, drop throughout the day, and are at their lowest in the middle of the night. A burst of cortisol between 6 and 8 a.m. wakes the brain from sleep and provides energy, and lower levels in the evening make us feel sleepy. If cortisol is too low, though, or if the pattern of release is abnormal, it leads to fatigue. Cortisol also controls how much glucose gets into the cells to be burned for energy, so if levels are too high or too low, the cells won't get enough energy, which also causes fatigue.

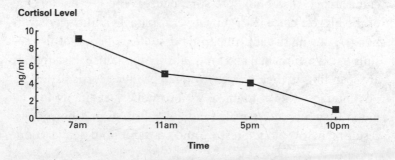

Normal pattern of cortisol secretion.

Adrenals in Fibromyalgia

In fibromyalgia the adrenal glands work hard. The continual bombardment of the stress response forces them to pump out cortisol continuously, resulting in overworked glands that never get to rest, because even at night the stress response signals keep them going. The result is adrenal burnout, a decrease in the glands' ability to carry out their normal functions. With long-term stress the adrenal glands can't secrete enough cortisol and develop abnormal functionality. Rats that are exposed to stress initially release high levels of cortisol, but if it persists for weeks, the levels drop as the adrenals burn out (Reber 2007).

To assess the function of the adrenal glands we have to look at the pattern of cortisol secretion over twenty-four hours. Any deviation from the normal cycle indicates strain on the adrenals. Most fibromyalgia patients show mild adrenal burnout, with a flattening of the usual curve of hormonal release throughout the day. Several studies have shown this "blunting" of the normal pattern of cortisol secretion in fibromyalgia patients (Mahdi 2011; Riedel 1998; Riva 2010).

Symptoms of Adrenal Burnout

In addition to fatigue, the symptoms of adrenal burnout include anxiety, low blood pressure, nausea, and low libido. One of the biggest clues is if you get very irritable and shaky when hungry. Losing the anti-inflammatory effect of cortisol also results in environmental and food sensitivities. Since the adrenals are spending all their energy trying to produce cortisol, there is not enough left over to make sex hormones, leading to low libido. They also don't make enough salt-retaining hormones, resulting in low blood pressure and constant mild dehydration.

Symptoms of Adrenal Burnout

- Fatigue
- Low blood pressure
- Feeling faint when standing up quickly
- Nausea
- Dizziness
- Severe anxiety
- Feeling shaky when you are hungry
- Feeling thirsty all the time
- Salt cravings
- Low libido
- Dark circles under the eyes
- Multiple food or environmental sensitivities
- Poor exercise tolerance

Diagnosing Adrenal Burnout

To diagnose adrenal burnout we need to look at the pattern of cortisol release by measuring levels in the saliva four times in a day, at 7 a.m., 11 a.m., 5 p.m., and 10 p.m. Saliva cortisol levels are at least as accurate as blood testing, and some experts think they are more reflective of the actual amounts of bioavailable hormone (Aardal 1995). Saliva tests can also measure levels of DHEA, a building-block hormone the adrenals use to make sex hormones. The amount of this building block indicates how well the adrenal glands are able to produces sex hormones. Low DHEA levels indicate more severe adrenal burnout.

Anytime the cortisol secretion cycle is abnormal it points to adrenal strain, but there are several possible patterns that indicate the severity or stage of burnout. In mild to moderate cases, we often see normal morning cortisol but with levels plummeting after noon. The more severe pattern reveals no morning spike and low levels all day. This flatline low indicates severely strained adrenals that have been drained of all their reserves and are struggling to produce enough cortisol to meet the body's demands. Another common pattern in cases of severe strain is low levels all day that spike at night (the exact opposite of what should be happening); these patients often experience insomnia.

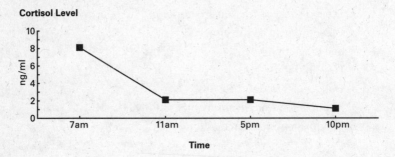

Mild/moderate adrenal burnout pattern.

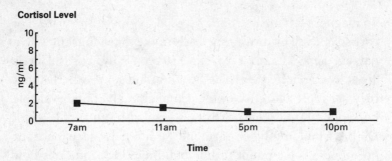

Severe adrenal burnout pattern.

But most doctors have never heard of or don't believe in the concept of subtle adrenal dysfunction like that seen in fibromyalgia. Conventional medicine measures cortisol levels only once in the morning, giving a snapshot that does not reveal the daily pattern. It often comes back in normal range, even in clear cases of adrenal burnout, since any of the four aberrant patterns may appear regular on a spot check. This type of test is only able to diagnose a complete adrenal shutdown, or "adrenal insufficiency," which can be life-threatening. It usually results from damage to the adrenals or to the part of the brain that controls the adrenal glands. Even in severe burnout the adrenals are still able to make cortisol, so it is not the same as adrenal insufficiency. If you think of the adrenals as a car, it can be running very low on gas but still be drivable. In adrenal insufficiency the gas tank is empty and the car won't move.

FAQ: Will adrenal burnout progress to adrenal insufficiency or adrenal shutdown?

No, complete adrenal shutdown is caused by injury to the adrenals by a virus or the immune system, or damage to the part of the brain that controls adrenal functioning. Being on high doses of prednisone or other steroids for many years can leave the adrenals in shutdown mode. But the adrenal burnout that we see in fibromyalgia does *not* progress to full adrenal shutdown. Instead, burned-out adrenals will limp along for a lifetime, but cause worsening fatigue over time.

Based on what I had learned in med school, I was initially quite skeptical that adrenal burnout even existed, but I became a convert once I saw so many of my patients benefit from treatment with naturopathic providers. If you are concerned that you may have adrenal burnout, I encourage you to talk to your HCP about getting salivary cortisol testing for an accurate diagnosis. Since many Western providers aren't trained in the concept, you may have more success working with a naturopath or holistic HCP for testing and treatment.

> ## FAQ: What if I can't find a provider who is willing to order the cortisol saliva testing for me?
>
> ---
>
> If you are not able to find a provider to work with you, there are several companies that offer testing directly to patients, but not all states allow patients to order the labs themselves. Even if you can order the test on your own, it is still preferable to work with a health care provider who can help you interpret the results and discuss treatment options.

Who Gets Severe Adrenal Burnout?

Although everyone with fibromyalgia has overworked adrenals, not everyone develops severe adrenal burnout. I see it more often in patients who in addition to fibromyalgia also have hypothyroidism or chronic fatigue syndrome, or are on long-term high-dose opiates. When thyroid hormone production is inadequate the adrenals often pick up the slack, so undertreated hypothyroidism can result in burnout. Chronic fatigue syndrome involves a continual activation of the immune response, which puts an additional burden on the adrenal glands and leads to more severe burnout.

Adrenal burnout commonly occurs in patients taking long-term high daily doses of opiate pain medications. High daily doses of opiates can interfere with the ability of adrenals to make cortisol (Oltmanns 2005; Pullan 1983; Müssig 2007; Merza 2010). For anyone with fibromyalgia who is taking opiates and experiencing extreme fatigue, I worry about adrenal burnout. See pages 215–216 for what is considered a high dose of opiates; it is generally above 120 mg of morphine daily (or the equivalent amount of another opiate).

Supporting the Overworked Adrenal Glands in Fibromyalgia

Everyone with fibromyalgia has overworked adrenal glands that need extra support. No matter what the stage of adrenal burnout, there are natural ways to support and improve their function. The Rest and Repair steps of getting more deep sleep, activating the relaxation response, and gentle exercise can help restore more normal patterns of cortisol secretion, and we can eat well, emphasize protein with every meal, and limit stimulants like caffeine, sugar, and alcohol. To perform, the adrenals need vitamins C, B_5, B_6, folic acid, magnesium, zinc, and copper. Folic acid can be hard for some people to process, so I recommend taking an activated form.

FAQ: How can I get more magnesium?

Magnesium supplements are the easiest way to get enough of the most important mineral for adrenal function. Some forms, magnesium oxide in particular, are not well absorbed from the intestines. Magnesium malate, citrate, and glycinate are the most usable forms. You can also absorb it through your skin by bathing with Epsom salt or using magnesium oils or lotions. Certain foods are also rich in magnesium, including dark chocolate, leafy green vegetables, nuts and seeds, bananas, and some types of mineral water.

Further support for the adrenals includes drinking plenty of water and increasing salt consumption, especially sea salt. One easy way to do this is by adding one-quarter teaspoon of sea salt to sixteen ounces of water and drinking twice daily (it should be dilute enough that it doesn't taste salty). Salt helps keeps fluid in your bloodstream to reduce that "peeing all the time but still thirsty" feeling that is so common in fibromyalgia. It also supplies needed minerals to the adrenal glands.

Salt can aggravate high blood pressure, so if you have that condition make sure to talk with your HCP first. Many patients with high blood pressure can't tolerate the added sea salt, so for them I recommend just supplementing with the other supportive vitamins and minerals.

Supporting Adrenal Glands

- Drink dilute sea-salt water.
- Supplement with vitamins C, B_5, and B_6.
- Take magnesium and zinc; they are the most important minerals.
- Take activated folic acid.
- Practice good sleep habits.
- Increase deep sleep.
- Do regular gentle exercise.
- Limit stimulants such as refined sugars and caffeine.
- Eat lots of protein.

FAQ: Can I just drink regular table salt in water?

No, it has to be natural sea salt. Regular table salt is just sodium, whereas sea salt includes other trace minerals including magnesium, zinc, copper, manganese, and sulfur. These minerals combined with the sodium are what help support the adrenal glands. Note that sea salt does not contain much iodine, which is important for thyroid health, so continue to use iodized table salt with food.

FAQ: What is activated folic acid?

Common genetic variations affect the body's ability to activate and use supplemental folic acid. L-5-methyl-tetrahydrofolate is the universally metabolized and active form, meaning it bypasses several enzymatic activation steps and is directly usable by the body, regardless of functional or genetic variations. I recommend reliable brands such as Thorne Research or Pure Encapsulations, in daily dosage of 400–800 mcg, to support adrenal health.

Treating Adrenal Burnout

Patients with severe adrenal burnout may need treatment beyond the supportive measures listed in the previous section. First, we must address anything else that may be interfering with adrenal function. High-dose opiates interfere with the adrenals' ability to make cortisol, so doses should be slowly lowered if possible. Under- or overtreated hypothyroidism can push the adrenals into hyperdrive and deplete them, so work with your HCP to make sure that your hypothyroidism is being adequately treated.

The next step is to try adaptogenic herbs, which improve the body's ability to cope with stress and can improve adrenal function. My two favorites are rhodiola and ashwagandha. *Rhodiola rosea* is a flowering plant that has been shown to reduce the stress response and reduce anxiety and fatigue (Olsson 2009; Panossian 2007; Ishaque 2012). In particular, supplementation of rhodiola helps patients with severe anxiety. The usual dosage is 100–200 mg daily. Ashwagandha (*Withania somnifera*) is an herb from the Indian Ayurvedic healing tradition that ameliorates the effects of stress in rats and humans (Bhattacharya 2003; Chandrasekhar 2012). The usual dosage is 150–300 mg daily.

FAQ: Does rhodiola have any side effects?

The main side effect is feeling overstimulated or jittery, which usually improves on a lower dosage. When I take rhodiola I have weird dreams, which my patients also commonly report. Usually this side effect gets better over time, and when supplements are taken in the morning and at lunch.

People with advanced adrenal burnout may need more aggressive treatment with adrenal glandular extracts and in the most severe cases even a short time on prescription hydrocortisone. Glandular supplements (extracts from liquid or powdered bovine adrenal glands) boost the functioning of the adrenals in humans by providing the essential building blocks for adrenal repair and concentrated nutrients in the forms needed for proper function. They are not replacement hormones and contain only tiny amounts of the actual hormones found in the adrenal glands. Iagen makes SR-Adrenal, which has many of the nutrients needed to support adrenals, along with rhodiola, ashwagandha, and adrenal glandular extract. Another good option is called a-Drenal, made by RLC Labs.

For patients who are demonstrating a reverse cortisol pattern—high cortisol levels in the evening—we need to restore a normal cycle. The best way is to supplement with phosphatidylserine (PS), a naturally occurring phospholipid nutrient that is most concentrated in organs with high metabolic activity, including the brain, liver, and skeletal muscle. PS modulates the cortisol-related activity of receptors and signaling molecules, and supplementation has been shown to lower cortisol levels (Hellhammer 2014; Starks 2008; Monteleone 1990, 1992). This is best taken one hour before the time(s) of day when cortisol levels are elevated. I like a supplement called Seriphos, which provides the activated form of phosphatidylserine.

I treat adrenal burnout with a combination of the above supplements for at least three months; they can be stopped once symptoms improve. Don't expect instant results—it usually takes at least a month before your fatigue will lessen. Cases of severe adrenal dysfunction may require six months to a year of this extra support. Treatment of adrenal fatigue can be complex, so I recommend consulting with a health care provider prior to taking any of these supplements. She can help you adjust your regimen as needed, and can also determine if prescription medication may be required.

Hydrocortisone for Severe Adrenal Burnout

For more severe cases of adrenal burnout, such as the flatline low levels seen in the figure on page 152, we may need to artificially supply cortisol to the body to take some pressure off the glands and give them time to reboot. Prescription hydrocortisone is identical to the natural form of cortisol and when administered at 20 mg per day emulates a normal daily cortisol secretion. Use of hydrocortisone is a temporary assist so the adrenal glands don't have to spend all their energy churning out cortisol, giving them an opportunity to recuperate and heal.

Administering hydrocortisone in this way is not accepted by most Western medical providers, as it runs the risk of causing the adrenal glands to shut down completely. However, this usually happens only at daily dosages of 20 mg or higher. No studies have looked at using hydrocortisone specifically for adrenal fatigue, but there is research on its effect on chronic fatigue syndrome. One found that 25–35 mg of hydrocortisone replacement for twenty-eight days improved fatigue in CFS, but follow-up blood testing showed it induced mild adrenal shutdown (McKenzie 1998). Another using a lower dose of 5–10 mg daily for one month showed fatigue reduction and no signs of adrenal shutdown (Cleare 1999). However, a third study showed no improvement in fatigue with 5 mg daily for three months (Blockmans 2003).

Because of the risk of adrenal shutdown, it is important to take daily doses of 15 mg or lower for six months or less, and only if all other treatments for adrenal burnout have not worked. For patients who also have hypothyroidism, I carefully monitor and adjust thyroid hormone replacement dosages, as cortisol enables more thyroid hormone to be absorbed into cells and can cause hyperthyroidism (excess thyroid hormone). If you have hypothyroidism it is essential to make sure to work with a health care provider on adrenal hormone balancing. The adrenal and thyroid hormones interact closely, and you will learn more about thyroid hormone in the next chapter.

To Do Yourself

- Bolster your adrenals by drinking water with sea salt, adding adrenal support vitamins and minerals, and engaging in gentle exercise.
- If you have mild adrenal burnout symptoms and do not have hypothyroidism or chronic fatigue syndrome, or take daily opiate pain medication, it is reasonable to get salivary testing on your own and take focused adrenal support supplements for a few month such as SR-Adrenal by Iagen (www.iagen.com) or a-Drenal by RLC Labs (www.rlclabs.com).
- **IMPORTANT: If you have hypothyroidism, please seek treatment from a naturopath or other integrative HCP before ordering saliva cortisol testing or starting any adrenal supplements.**
- To get salivary cortisol testing done direct from a lab (in most states, you're able to order without a doctor's prescription), contact Genova Diagnostics (www.gdx.net) or ZRT Laboratory (www. zrtlab.com) and order an adrenal stress profile.

To Discuss with Your Health Care Provider

- If you have symptoms of severe adrenal burnout, chronic fatigue syndrome, or hypothyroidism, or take daily opiate pain medications, I advise working closely with a health care provider to manage adrenal support protocols.

CHAPTER 16

Rebalance: Thyroid and Sex Hormones

In the last chapter you learned about the strain that fibromyalgia can put on the adrenal glands. Remember, the adrenals are the foundation of your hormonal house, and if they are out of whack it will cause imbalances in the thyroid and sex hormones as well. It's all related. For example, a frequent cause of persistent fatigue in fibromyalgia is undiagnosed or undertreated hypothyroidism. Low or fluctuating levels of sex hormones in both men and women also worsen fibromyalgia symptoms.

Often, improving adrenal function restores balance to the thyroid and sex hormones. But in some cases, especially in people who have both hypothyroidism and fibromyalgia, we may need to focus more specifically on the thyroid. One study found that 31 percent of patients with hypothyroidism also had fibromyalgia, and patients with both diseases report higher levels of pain and fatigue than those with fibromyalgia alone (Soy 2007; Bazzichi 2007).

The Gray Zone of Hypothyroidism and Fibromyalgia

Let me be clear: hypothyroidism does not cause fibromyalgia, and not everyone with fibromyalgia has hypothyroidism. But for patients with both, it can be difficult to establish whether it is their low levels of thyroid hormone that are causing fatigue, as there is major overlap in the symptoms of these two conditions, including fatigue, depression, and poor memory. But there are some things that only occur with hypothyroidism and point to a diminished thyroid as a source of fatigue.

Distinguishing Symptoms of Hypothyroidism

- Dry skin and hair
- Hair loss
- Thinning eyebrows at the outer portion
- Unexplained weight gain or difficulty losing weight
- Irregular menstrual periods
- Puffiness and swelling around the eyes, hands, and feet
- Feeling cold when others are not
- Constipation

Having fibromyalgia can make getting an accurate diagnosis of and effective treatment for hypothyroidism much, much harder. Western doctors tend to have a very black-and-white view of hypothyroidism and base diagnosis and treatment decisions solely on one lab value. But when it occurs alongside fibromyalgia this number can be misleading. Getting the right tests and treatment for hypothyroidism can make a huge difference in fatigue for patients stuck in this gray zone.

What Is Hypothyroidism, Anyway?

The thyroid gland sits at the base of your neck, just above your collarbone, and secretes hormones in response to chemical signals from the brain. In hypothyroidism, it simply does not make enough.

Thyroid hormones control how quickly your cells burn

energy—your metabolism. If you don't have enough, your body processes slow down, you feel cold all the time, and you don't process calories efficiently. Your skin and hair become dry and unhealthy. Your bowels slow down and become constipated. The most common cause is Hashimoto's thyroiditis, an autoimmune disease in which the body produces antibodies that attack and destroy the thyroid gland.

The hypothalamus in the brain directs the activity of the thyroid gland by telling the pituitary gland to make thyroid-stimulating hormone (TSH). TSH travels in the blood to the thyroid and stimulates hormone production, of which there are two types: T3 and T4. T4 is the main hormone produced by the thyroid, but it is really a pre-hormone because it must be converted by our cells into the active form T3 before it can be used.

To diagnose hypothyroidism, doctors usually look for an elevated TSH. When thyroid hormone is too low in the body, the brain will start pumping out TSH to increase the levels. So if the thyroid is not making enough hormone, TSH levels will be abnormally high as the brain frantically tries to signal the thyroid to boost production. To treat hypothyroidism, patients are usually given synthetic replacement of T4, a prescription called levothyroxine (Synthroid). It's considered a fairly straightforward diagnosis and treatment.

Fibromyalgia muddies the waters and makes it harder to accurately diagnose hypothyroidism. The hypothalamus—the same area of the brain that controls the stress response—also directs the release of thyroid hormones. Chronic hyperactivity of the stress response affects signaling between the brain and the thyroid, resulting in a diminished TSH reaction to low thyroid hormone. HCPs look for an elevated TSH to diagnose hypothyroidism, but the blunted TSH response in fibromyalgia means that TSH can be normal even if thyroid hormone levels are low. Doctors can miss a hypothyroidism diagnosis if they rely on TSH alone; they need to check T3 and T4 levels as well (Riedel 1998). Even if the TSH is fine, if T4 or T3 are low and there are ongoing hypothyroid-specific symptoms, a diagnosis of hypothyroidism is appropriate.

Treating Hypothyroidism in Fibromyalgia

Treating hypothyroidism in fibromyalgia is tricky and has to take into account that most everyone with fibromyalgia has some adrenal burnout and also may have an impaired ability to convert thyroid hormone into its active form. Adrenal burnout must be addressed first, because if the adrenals are not functioning well, thyroid hormone won't be taken up into cells, resulting in persistent symptoms of hypothyroidism. Think of cortisol as the key that opens the door to let thyroid hormone into the cells; it also helps translate thyroid hormone into its active form. Either low or high levels of cortisol can interfere with the conversion of T4 to T3.

Fibromyalgia patients who are not responding adequately to thyroid replacement often have burnt-out adrenal glands that are not producing enough cortisol. Thyroid hormones can't function inside a cell if there is not enough cortisol to transport them inside. Michelle, my patient going through the nasty divorce, was on the correct dosage of thyroid replacement according to her labs but was still profoundly fatigued and having persistent hypothyroid symptoms. Once we addressed her adrenal glands, her fatigue lifted and her eyebrows started growing back!

Furthermore, the typical treatment of hypothyroidism with T4 replacement alone may not be adequate, because a constant hyperactive stress response can block conversion of T4 to the active form T3 (Tsigos 2002). (Even people without fibromyalgia can have problems converting T4 into T3.) One study found that 16 percent of patients with hypothyroidism had a genetic variation for a less active enzyme that converts T4 to T3, and they tended to feel better when taking a combination of both T3 and T4, rather than T4 alone (Panicker 2009).

I see many patients with fibromyalgia and hypothyroidism who are taking enough T4 (levothyroxine) but still have severe fatigue and other classic symptoms of low thyroid. Their T4 and TSH lab values will often be normal, because the hypothalamus is sensing that there is enough T4 in the bloodstream. But since not enough T4 is being converted into usable T3, their cells are still not getting enough of the hormone—so I always make sure to test for T3.

I will often prescribe low levels of T3 (liothyronine) in addition to the T4 to compensate for a diminished ability to convert T4 to T3. T3 has a shorter half-life than T4 so is usually dosed twice daily. T3 has made a huge difference for my patients suffering from undertreated hypothyroidism. The key is keeping doses low, because at higher levels it can cause anxiety or jitteriness.

Another option is a medication made from pig thyroid gland that contains both T4 and T3 (the most common brand is Armour). In one study, nearly half of the participants felt better on the dried pig thyroid than T4 alone (Hoang 2013). Because it is not an accepted treatment, this type of medication may not be covered by insurance. With either method it is important to closely monitor for symptoms of excess thyroid hormone, which include heart palpitations and rapid bone loss leading to osteoporosis.

Daily Recommended Thyroid Support Nutrients

Selenium 200–400 mcg

Zinc 15–30 mg

Vitamin D 2,000 IU

Vitamin A 2,000 IU

Iodine 150 mcg

Iron supplementation to achieve a ferritin of 50–100

Thyroid Support Nutrients

You can also support your body's ability to convert T4 to the active form T3 with nutrients. Selenium, zinc, iron, and iodine are all minerals used synergistically by the thyroid to produce its hormones (Zimmermann 2002). Unfortunately, due to soil mineral depletion many diets are deficient in these nutrients. The enzyme that converts T4 to T3 needs selenium, and people with low-selenium diets have a reduced ability to create the active T3 (Olivieri 1996). Mice fed a diet low in selenium and zinc had lower T4 and T3 levels compared to mice on their normal diet; they also had lower levels of the enzyme that converts between the two forms (Kralik 1996). Finally, iron deficiency impairs thyroid hormone production, so it is important to get checked if you have hypothyroidism. The most sensitive marker for iron stores in the body is ferritin, and although a low ferritin is considered to be 10 or below, the range for optimal thyroid function is 50–100. Vitamins A and D also support healthy thyroid function.

My recommendations for support nutrients for optimal thyroid function are listed above, and remember that they work synergistically, especially iodine and selenium; that is, you shouldn't take iodine without also taking selenium. I've also listed some thyroid support supplement complexes at the end of the chapter that include most of these nutrients. High levels of inflammation also interfere with the body's ability to utilize thyroid hormones, and one of the most common hidden culprits is sensitivity to foods, especially gluten. If you have hypothyroidism, I always recommend at least an eight-week trial of a gluten-free diet to see if you notice any improvement in fatigue.

Alternative Versus Conventional Treatment of Hypothyroidism

The treatment of hypothyroidism is probably the biggest area in medicine where naturopaths and Western doctors disagree. Administering dried pig thyroid, or even T3 in addition to the usual T4, remains controversial. The American Thyroid Association 2014 guidelines advocate T4 *only* for treatment of hypothyroidism, and most Western doctors don't prescribe pig thyroid gland due to concerns about a stable dosage, as ratios of T4 to T3 can vary from 5:1 to 2:1 in pig thyroid products. In fact, the prescribing handbook used by most Western medicine doctors lists Armour Thyroid as "obsolete" and strongly discourages its use.

Naturopaths often treat hypothyroidism by adjusting the hormone replacement based on patient symptoms rather than focusing on the labs, whereas the conventional approach is to modify hormones based strictly on TSH levels, not specific symptoms, and to only use T4 replacement. For example, if a thyroid replacement medication brings a patient's TSH back to the normal range, even if the patient is still having low thyroid symptoms, a Western medicine doctor would not make any further dosage adjustments. But in this same case a naturopath might increase T4 further or add a low dose of T3, or change to a pig thyroid product that contains both T3 and T4.

Since the chronic stress response in fibromyalgia can interfere with thyroid lab tests and impair conversion of T4 to active form T3, it is especially important to closely monitor the full panel of thyroid labs, including T4, T3, and TSH. I have found that for subtle adjustment of thyroid hormones or for more detailed testing, a naturopathic perspective can be helpful. If you are concerned about undiagnosed or undertreated hypothyroidism, consider seeing a naturopath or holistic HCP.

Sex Hormones

The sex hormones, testosterone, estrogen, and progesterone, can get thrown off balance in fibromyalgia, exacerbating its symptoms. Nearly half of menstruating women with fibromyalgia reported a worsening of pain and fatigue during menses (Pamuk 2005). About a quarter of patients feel their symptoms got worse during or after menopause (Pamuk 2005).

Since adrenals form the foundation of your hormonal house, adrenal burnout affects the equilibrium of the sex hormones. Often, restoring adrenal function will lessen those symptoms, so we start there. I have observed that women suffering from worsened fibromyalgia symptoms due to menopause often have adrenal burnout—and studies back this up. Severity of PMS has also been linked to adrenal dysfunction (Woods 1998). Menopausal women with more severe fibromyalgia symptoms also have lower DHEA levels, a marker of adrenal health. So if you are struggling with worsened fibromyalgia symptoms during certain times of the menstrual cycle or menopause, first focus on improving the health of your adrenal glands (Miller 2013).

If adrenal balancing doesn't help, sex hormone replacement therapy is an option. For some women, hormone replacement alleviates the worsening of their symptoms during menopause; for others, it does not. If menopausal night sweats or hot flashes are disturbing your sleep, hormone replacement can give you relief and improve sleep quality (Gambacciani 2005). In my clinical experience I have seen patients improve on hormones, but the one study that has been done concluded that estrogen replacement does not improve fibromyalgia pain in post-menopausal women (Stening 2011). The intensification of symptoms that occurs as hormones transition to the lower levels seen in menopause is temporary, usually lasting about a year or two. Since hormone replacement therapy increases the risk of breast and uterine cancer, the safest approach is to wait it out. However, if you have already maximized support to your adrenal glands and are still struggling with higher levels of pain and fatigue or disturbed sleep in early menopause, it may be worth talking with your HCP about hormone replacement therapy.

FAQ: Are bioidentical hormones safer?

Many prescription replacements are chemicals that are similar, but not identical, to the estrogen and progesterone made by the body. Bioidentical hormones are interchangeable with those that are made and metabolized in the human female body. They tend to be better tolerated and may confer fewer cancer risks than synthetic hormones (L'hermite 2008; Holtorf 2009). Bioidentical hormone prescriptions are just estradriol and progesterone, the same hormones made by the body. Topical formulations are thought to be the safest, and include patches or custom-compounded creams.

For men with fibromyalgia, low testosterone levels will exacerbate their symptoms (Traish 2009). As men age, testosterone production naturally drops, but my male patients tend to have lower testosterone than expected for their age group. However, it is not clear that all men with fibromyalgia have lower levels—one small study found no difference in levels compared to healthy men (Yoshikawa 2010). A complicating factor is that many men with fibromyalgia are on opiate pain medication, which suppresses testosterone—one study found that 74 percent of men on high-dose opioids had low levels of the hormone (Smith 2012; Daniell 2002).

Symptoms of Low Testosterone

- Lack of energy
- Lethargy
- Sadness/grumpiness
- Diminished muscle mass and weakness
- Decreased strength and endurance
- Erection weakness
- Decreased libido

Replacement therapy with creams, gels, pellets, or injections increases muscle mass and strength and improves exercise endurance and balance (Brill 2002). I have found that it reduces fatigue and muscle pain in my male patients with low testosterone. However, as with hormone replacement therapy for women, the jury is still out about its long-term safety. Some studies show that testosterone replacement increases a man's risk of heart attack and stroke, while others report that it is protective and *reduces* the risk of heart attack and stroke (Vigen 2013; Xu 2013; Malkin 2010; Schwarz 2011). It may also increase the risk of prostate cancer, although several large studies showed no danger (Roddam 2008; Rhoden 2004). If you do go on testosterone, you should screen for prostate cancer before and during treatment.

The safest approach to restoring balance to your testosterone is to support the adrenal glands. If high-dose opiates are suppressing hormonal production, reducing or stopping them will allow those levels to come up. And as if easing your symptoms across the board wasn't enough, exercise also stimulates testosterone release (Hough 2011). But if all these measures fail, talk to your HCP about getting tested for low testosterone and possible treatment with replacement therapy.

- Make sure you are supporting your adrenal glands (chapter 15).

If you have hypothyroidism and fibromyalgia:

- Try going gluten free for two months.
- Take a high-quality thyroid support supplement that contains selenium, iodine, and zinc. I recommend Thyroid Support Complex by Pure Encapsulations or Thyrocsin from Thorne Research.
- Consider seeing a naturopathic or holistic physician for specialized help managing hypothyroidism.

To Discuss with Your Health Care Provider

- Ask your HCP to check T4 and T3 levels in addition to TSH levels.
- If you are concerned about undiagnosed or undertreated hypothyroidism, consider seeing a naturopath or holistic HCP.
- If you are a man with symptoms of low testosterone, ask about getting your levels checked.
- If you are a woman with menopause-related worsening of fibromyalgia symptoms, ask about hormone replacement therapy.

_____

CHAPTER 17

Rebalance: Mood

That's the worst thing about depression: A human being can survive almost anything as long as she sees the end in sight. But depression is so insidious, and it compounds daily, that it's impossible to ever see the end. The fog is like a cage without a key.
—ELIZABETH WURTZEL

The steps you have already taken to lower inflammation and balance your hormones will help your mood as well. Elevated levels of inflammatory chemicals are known to worsen depression, as do hormonal imbalances such as low thyroid and adrenal burnout (Tsao 2006; Krueger 2011). So I hope you're already feeling better, but now is the time to address any remaining mood issues. It is vital to restore your emotional balance; mood disorders can be paralyzing and interfere with your ability to take action.

Let's face it—being in pain is depressing. And if you're in a pit of depression or paralyzed by anxiety it's nearly impossible to do anything to help yourself feel better. Not only does being in pain affect every aspect of your emotional and physical life, but it actually causes changes to brain structure and function, activating the areas associated with depression (Gustin 2013). Chronic pain also shifts the balance in your brain's chemicals toward those associated with anxiety and depression. For example, researchers have found that "chronic back pain alters the human brain chemistry" (Grachev 2000). The good news is that our brains have "neuronal plasticity"—that is, with proper training, they can learn new ways to connect and develop new patterns. Diet, exercise, and prescription medications and supplements can all alter our brain chemistry for the better.

Compared to other chronic illnesses, fibromyalgia is more often accompanied by depression, anxiety, and post-traumatic stress disorder (PTSD). One report found that 60 percent of subjects with fibromyalgia met the criteria for major depression, compared to 28 percent of rheumatoid arthritis patients (Walker 1997). Survivors of trauma suffer from much higher rates of depression and anxiety than the general population, and many develop PTSD (Maes 2000). Most people diagnosed with fibromyalgia have suffered a major trauma; in fact, 90 percent of women with fibromyalgia reported being physically or sexually assaulted in their lifetime (Walker 1997).

Western medicine is very skilled at managing most mood disorders, so I encourage you to talk openly about these issues with your HCP. I like to take an integrative approach and utilize the most effective treatments from both alternative and conventional medicine. This chapter reviews the integrative treatments I have found effective to treat depression, anxiety, and PTSD in people with fibromyalgia.

Depression

Not everyone with fibromyalgia is clinically depressed, and depression does *not* cause fibromyalgia. But if depression occurs in conjunction with fibromyalgia it can make it much harder for you to help yourself with movement therapy or diet changes.

Depression is characterized by a flattened mood and feelings of worthlessness or guilt. A depressed person feels markedly diminished interest or pleasure in almost all activities and may have recurring thoughts of death or suicide. It's a complex condition related to brain biochemistry, genetics, and life stressors. The part of the brain that experiences pain is located right next to the part that regulates mood, and there is a great deal of overlap. That is, pain can make depression worse, and depression can make pain worse. Most HCPs are well equipped to treat depression with prescription antidepressants. Some increase both serotonin and norepinephrine levels, such as duloxetine (Cymbalta), milnacipran (Savella), and venlafaxine (Effexor), which can improve mood and pain simultaneously.

But for some patients prescription antidepressants only partially work. For them, I have found the addition of a specialized folic acid supplement to be helpful. Some people don't produce enough of an enzyme (MTHFR) that converts folic acid into the active form—L-methylfolate—that the brain uses to make mood-enhancing chemicals, especially serotonin. Those with genes that code for dysfunctional folate-converting enzymes are not able to produce as much of the active form of folic acid, and are more likely to suffer from depression. In fact, one study found that 70 percent of depressed patients had a gene for a dysfunctional MTHFR enzyme (Kelly 2004; Lewis 2006). Problems with the MTHFR gene have also been connected to an increased risk of stroke and heart attack.

FAQ: Should I get tested for the MTHFR mutation?

There are about forty known genetic mutations that code for a dysfunctional MTHFR enzyme, but only two that are commonly tested for, C677T and A129C. The former is the most serious and most studied mutation. If you are heterozygous (meaning you have one abnormal gene and one normal gene) you will have a 30 percent reduction in folate production. If you are homozygous for C677T (two copies of the abnormal gene), that goes up to 70 percent. It is worth getting tested if you have any risk factors, like a family history of early stroke or heart attack. However, you do not necessarily need to get tested only for depression, as the test is expensive and may not be covered by insurance. I often will just try the activated form of folate to see if it helps mood.

Depression can be eased by supplementing the diet with the activated form of folic acid. For patients who are on an antidepressant but need some extra help, I give them prescription L-methylfolate (Deplin). L-methylfolate bypasses the MTHFR enzyme altogether so that the activated folic acid can enter the brain, where it is turned into mood-lifting chemicals like serotonin. Several studies have shown improvement in depression with L-methylfolate alone, or in combination with other antidepressants (Coppen 2000; Passeri 1993; Godfrey 1990). I've seen great results in some patients with severe depression by

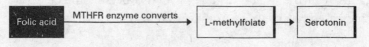

Conversion of folic acid.

adding this supplement in addition to antidepressant medications. The recommended dosage is 15 mg daily, and it may take three to four weeks before you see an effect (Miller 2008).

Another option is the supplement 5-hydroxytryptophan (5-HTP), which your body converts into serotonin. When combined with other serotonin-increasing medications like antidepressants, it can cause serotonin excess, which can be toxic and lead to serotonin syndrome. Symptoms range from shivering and diarrhea to muscle rigidity, fever and seizures, and even death if it isn't treated. (For more information on this syndrome see page 78). If you currently take antidepressants, talk with your HCP before trying 5-HTP.

FAQ: Is L-methylfolate the same as L-5-methyltetrahydrofolate?

They are both the activated form of folic acid that the brain can use, but they differ slightly in their chemical composition. L-methylfolate (Deplin) is stronger and available only by prescription. It has also been the most studied. L-5-methyltetrahydrofolate is available without a prescription but is not as powerful. If you do choose the over-the-counter version I recommend reliable brands such as Thorne Research or Pure Encapsulations.

Anxiety

The emotional experience of a stress response system that is on red alert all the time is often one of anxiety or panic. In addition to the physical symptoms of fibromyalgia, many sufferers report a generalized feeling of unease or "just never feeling safe." This is directly related, in my opinion, to the emotional experience of a brain forever ready for fight or flight.

The most common prescription for anxiety is benzodiazepines, but as you read in chapter 8, these medications interfere with deep sleep and are not ideal in fibromyalgia. If you must take benzodiazepines for anxiety, try to keep them away from sleep hours as much as possible to limit negative side effects. I also urge you to try other ways to manage anxiety.

The tools you learned in the Rest chapters to mitigate the effects of the stress response will also reduce anxiety. The flowering plant rhodiola has been very effective for many of my patients, and studies confirm that it can reduce anxiety (Ishaque 2012). The usual dosage is 100 mg two to three times daily. Another approach used by some holistic providers is prescription sublingual oxytocin, a brain chemical that modulates attachment and social behaviors. It is released naturally in the brain after orgasm and childbirth and has been called the "bonding" hormone. It may also help reduce anxiety (Dodhia 2014; Labuschagne 2010; Kirsch 2005).

Non-Benzodiazepine Anxiety Treatments

- Relaxation response
- Rhodiola supplement
- Oxytocin
- Beta-blockers
- Buspirone
- Antidepressants—SSRIs
- Gabapentin

There are also effective prescriptions for anxiety out there, in particular medications that increase serotonin in the brain. The serotonin-boosting (selective serotonin reuptake inhibitor, or SSRI) antidepressants include fluoxetine (Prozac) and sertraline (Zoloft). Buspirone (Buspar) is not an SSRI but also works on serotonin receptors in the brain, and I've seen some great results. You've already heard about gabapentin for its positive effects on sleep; it can also help anxiety (Lavigne 2012). The usual dosage for anxiety is 100–300 mg twice daily. Another option is low doses of the beta-blockers pindolol or propranolol (Khadke 2012; Dyck 1991). These medications lower blood pressure and slow heart rate, and so must be used cautiously, but they are a good choice if you suffer from high blood pressure in addition to anxiety.

Post-Traumatic Stress Disorder (PTSD)

About a quarter of people with fibromyalgia also have posttraumatic stress disorder. PTSD is an anxiety disorder characterized by nightmares, recurrent memories of traumatic events, and avoidance behaviors (Arnold 2004). Nightmares, of course, can be very disruptive to sleep, so treatment is paramount. One option is a medication called an alpha-blocker, taken at bedtime, which blocks some of the fight-or-flight and fear responses in the brain. I generally use the alpha-blocker prazosin since it has been thoroughly studied and found to be effective for PTSD (Taylor 2008).

PTSD Symptom Survey

Have you had any experience that was so frightening, horrible, or upsetting that *in the past month* you:
- Had nightmares about it?
- Went out of your way to avoid situations that reminded you of it?
- Were constantly on guard, watchful, or easily startled?
- Felt numb or detached from others, activities, or your surroundings?

If you answered yes to one or more, talk with your HCP about PTSD.

Another option is psychotherapy. One of the more effective techniques is eye movement desensitization and reprocessing (EMDR), in which the patient thinks and talks about the trauma while tracking the therapist's finger as it moves back and forth across her visual field. The theory is that the side-to-side eye movement helps the brain process the emotions associated with trauma (Cloitre 2009).

I like to address the emotional manifestations of trauma by taking an energetic approach. The theory here is that a trauma, accident, or attack on your physical body leaves an imprint on your energy field. A patient who had been sexually abused by her brother told me she always felt as if "he was under my skin." These energetic signatures of trauma exist outside the speech and thought centers of the brain, and thus are difficult to access with traditional talk therapy. There are various techniques a practitioner will use to manipulate a patient's energy and remove the energetic imprint of trauma. First, she will usually interpret the patient's energy fields and then remove any perceived dysfunctional energy with her own movement or intention. This can be subtle and not physically felt by the client, or instantly palpable.

I might be skeptical if I hadn't experienced stunning results myself. At my first visit with an energy healer we talked briefly about the sexual assault I suffered in adolescence. After asking my permisson, she placed one hand on my thigh and one on my stomach. She told me to tell my attacker's energy to leave my body. It felt ridiculous but I said it aloud. After a few minutes I began to feel waves of something similar to nausea, like pulses of energy coming up from my stomach. I almost gagged, and then I was spewing what felt like his energy up and out of my mouth, vomiting him up and out of me. I felt as if I was convulsing in spasms—but I wasn't moving at all.

Afterward I felt so much lighter and quieter, it was like when you hear the whirring noise of the fridge stop. While it's running you don't even notice it, but when it stops you become acutely aware of the quiet and calm it leaves. I worked with this therapist for several more treatments and the whole experience was life-altering. It left me stronger, calmer, and happier.

That experience piqued my curiosity, so I hit the textbooks and attended several training sessions with experts in the field. I learned that the movement of electricity within our bodies does indeed create subtle biomagnetic fields that extend about three feet around us and can be measured with sensitive instruments. Stronger energy fields have been found to emanate from the hands of energy healers as compared to control subjects, providing support for the idea that humans can learn to direct or channel it (Zimmerman 1990; Seto 1992). Trust me: I know it sounds really out there and woo-woo (I shudder to think what my med school professors would say), but I have seen it bring powerful emotional healing and restore balance to many people suffering from the aftereffects of trauma.

My science brain still can't quite understand exactly how energy healing works. But after experiencing such profound benefits personally, I realized that just because I can't understand something doesn't mean that it is not real or true. One example is infrared light, which is not visible to the naked eye. We can't usually see infrared light unless we put on special night-vision goggles. Perhaps some people have developed lenses to "see" and even manipulate energy? One scientist studying energy healing compares it to any other sense that humans can develop—an oenophile, for example, who has developed their palate to the point of detecting very subtle distinctions between wines that to the average person all taste the same (Oschman 2000).

Manual therapies are another way to release the energy of trauma, because they can unlock the signatures that are stuck in the body. Rosalyn Bruyere, a famous teacher of energy healing, says, "The issue is in the tissue." In particular, the fascia is thought to be a storehouse for emotional energy. Many myofascial release practitioners describe the discharge of emotions and memories during bodywork sessions. John F. Barnes, who developed myofascial release, says that when people experience trauma sometimes part of their energy leaves the body to survive that moment. In some myofascial release sessions, the therapist might encourage you to invite your own energy back in.

One of the definitions of healing is "to become whole again," and if you feel like that's what you need, I encourage you to seek out a practitioner. Energy work or myofascial release might not be right for you, but please pursue whatever path feels right to heal from the emotional and spiritual damage that trauma can inflict.

To Do Yourself

- For further reading on energy healing, check out *Wheels of Light: Chakras, Auras, and the Healing Energy of the Body* by Rosalyn Bruyere, and *Afterwards, You're a Genius: Faith, Medicine, and the Metaphysics of Healing* by Chip Brown.
- To find a myofascial release practitioner, visit www .mfrtherapists.com.

To Discuss with Your Health Care Provider

- If you have persistent depression while on an antidepressant, ask about a prescription for L-methylfolate (Deplin). If your insurance does not cover it, send the prescription to Brand Direct Health pharmacy for a reduced cash price: www.branddirecthealth.com.

- Ask about risks before taking 5-HTP, especially if you are already on prescription antidepressants.
- See if you should try a non-benzodiazepine treatment for anxiety.
- If you answered yes to any of the PTSD survey questions, ask about a referral to a mental health specialist for diagnosis and treatment.

CHAPTER 18

Reduce: Fatigue and Fibrofog

The best way to improve fatigue in fibromyalgia is to increase the restorative deep sleep you get each night. It can take time to find the right combination of medications and lifestyle changes, but once we do I usually observe a substantial decrease in fatigue. This is why we start by focusing on improving deep sleep, and next on supporting cellular energy production. Hopefully, you've also rebalanced any hormonal sources of fatigue like adrenal burnout or undertreated hypothyroidism. But even after Resting, Repairing, and Rebalancing, there may be residual fatigue. Perhaps it's due to the sedating side effects of medications used to treat pain, so shifting those medications away from daytime hours or stopping them altogether can help. As a last resort, a stimulant like one used to treat attention deficit disorder (ADD) can lessen fatigue as well. For patients with both fibromyalgia and chronic fatigue syndrome, treating the fatigue brought on by CFS may require a different approach; see chapter 23 for my recommendations.

The fatigue in fibromyalgia is often accompanied by poor concentration and memory problems, commonly referred to as "fibrofog." The medical term is "dyscognition," which means impaired mental processing. This can be the most disabling of fibromyalgia symptoms, and usually manifests as difficulty finding the right words, and problems multitasking. In one study, 88 percent of subjects reported cognitive dysfunction, with at least some limitations in concentration, making decisions, thinking, and memory (Schaefer 2011). Patients also perform poorly on certain tests of cognitive function, in particular evaluations of short-term memory and completing tasks while distracted; these impairments in memory mimic about twenty years of aging (Leavitt 2006; Park 2001). Fibrofog is due primarily to a lack of deep sleep and poor energy production in the brain, so the same steps taken in Rest and Repair will improve symptoms. Increasing blood flow to the brain, certain medications and supplements, and brain-training games can also help clear the fog.

Reduce Daytime Sedating Medications

Unfortunately, many of the medications used to treat fibromyalgia pain have side effects of sedation and sleepiness. The most sedating medications are pregabalin (Lyrica), gabapentin (Neurontin), and the muscle relaxants. To avoid daytime sleepiness, I will prescribe those medications to be taken only at night, or at much lower doses during the day. I often see patients who are on the maximum dosage of gabapentin (1,200 mg three times a day) and are basically sleepwalking through life. In this case, the simple change of reducing gabapentin to 300 mg in the morning, 600 mg in afternoon, and 1,200 mg at bedtime will reduce daytime sleepiness but still relieve pain.

If you are taking any of the medications listed here and have significant daytime sleepiness and fatigue, talk with your HCP about either reducing your daytime dosage or stopping the medication altogether to see if fatigue improves. High dosages of opiate-based pain medications can also be sedating, so some patients feel less fatigued after a similar daytime dosage reduction.

Sedating Medications Commonly Used to Treat Fibromyalgia Pain

pregabalin (Lyrica)

gabapentin (Neurontin)

cyclobenzaprine (Flexeril)

tizanidine (Zanaflex)

metaxalone (Skelaxin)

methocarbamol (Robaxin)

carisoprodol (Soma)

baclofen (Lioresal)

high-dose opiates

Stimulant Medications to Fight Fatigue

If all other measures fail, stimulant medications can help some patients. You are probably already familiar with the most common non-prescription stimulant: caffeine. Prescription stimulants are mostly derived from amphetamines and include amphetamine/dextroamphetamine (Adderall) and methylphenidate (Ritalin). They make you feel more alert and less fatigued by binding to receptors for the activating chemicals dopamine and norepinephrine in the brain. But they are also associated with side effects like anxiety, elevated heart rate, and increases in blood pressure, and can be addictive. If I prescribe these medications, I keep the doses very low. To avoid a negative impact on sleep I also avoid dosing after noon and in long-acting or extended-release forms.

The newer stimulants modafinil (Provigil) and armodafinil (Nuvigil) work in a different way than the classic amphetamine-like medications. They promote alertness by arousing the parts of the brain that control wakefulness and are much safer than the amphetamine-derived medications, as they aren't addictive, although they can still increase anxiety, insomnia, and hypertension. Modafinil and armodafinil are prescribed to treat the daytime sleepiness caused by narcolepsy and obstructive sleep apnea. Several reports have shown that modafinil and armodafinil can improve fatigue in fibromyalgia, but no large clinical trials have been done yet. Patients have reported that this type of medication reduces their fatigue and allows them to be more functional during the day (Schwartz 2007, 2010; Schaller 2001; Pachas 2003). Both are expensive and not usually covered by insurance to treat fibromyalgia-related fatigue, but if you also have obstructive sleep apnea they may be covered, since they are FDA-approved for that purpose.

Certain amino acids (protein building blocks) called branched-chain amino acids can also mitigate fatigue (Greer 2011). They work by blocking the absorption of tryptophan, one of the main chemicals that causes the brain to sense fatigue (and briefly acknowledged every Thanksgiving). These amino acids include leucine, isoleucine, and valine and can be supplemented at 1,200–3,000 mg per day, in divided doses, between meals. This kind of amino acid also reduces muscle damage during exercise, so can relieve fibromyalgia muscles that are working hard even while at rest (Greer 2007).

Ways to Reduce Fibromyalgia Fatigue

- Improve quality of sleep.
- Support cellular energy production.
- Treat adrenal burnout.
- Reduce or remove daytime sedating meds.
- Try stimulant medications.
- Take branched-chain amino acid supplements.

Clearing Fibrofog

Several factors contribute to fibrofog. A lack of deep sleep certainly leads to impaired cognition; healthy people who are sleep-deprived score very similarly to people with fibromyalgia on tests of memory and attention. Also, a brain that is distracted by pain can't pay as close attention to anything else. Fibromyalgia patients demonstrate decreased blood flow in areas of the brain important for cognition and increased blood flow in pain-processing areas (Glass 2011).

The best way that I have found to ease fibrofog is to improve the amount and quality of deep sleep. But there are some other ways to help as well. The brain, just like any organ, thrives on blood flow, so any exercise that pushes more to the brain can improve its function. Studies show that people who exercise regularly are less likely to develop dementia, and people with fibromyalgia perform better on cognitive tests after doing several months of regular exercise (Jedrziewski 2010; Munguía-Izquierdo 2007; Etnier 2009). The gentle movement therapy you started in the Repair section will get the blood flowing to your brain and promote memory and cognition.

Many people with fibromyalgia have very low blood pressure (under 100/60). To make sure your brain is getting enough blood, blood pressure should ideally be 120–140/60–90. Persistent low blood pressure means that the brain is not getting enough blood perfusion, which can worsen its performance. To naturally raise blood pressure, increase salt and water in your diet. Medications such as fludrocortisone (Florinef) can also increase your blood pressure. If you are on blood-pressure-lowering medications for hypertension, make sure you're not getting too low; signs include getting dizzy or faint when standing up. I'd also highly encourage you to buy a monitor for home use so you can keep an eye on your blood pressure. Often insurance will pay for these with a prescription. If your blood pressure is too low, talk with your HCP about adjusting your medications.

Building up the "muscles" of the brain is another effective way to clear the fog. Using a cognitive training video game, researchers were able to improve the ability of older adults to multitask (Abbott 2013). The most exciting finding was that improvements in brain performance were not seen just while playing the game but in other cognitive tasks. Check out the website Lumosity for games designed to improve your cognitive abilities.

Another treatment is giving your brain a zap of energy with low-dose electricity or light therapy. Cranial electrotherapy stimulation (CES) is microcurrent electricity transmitted through the brain between electrodes placed on each ear. It has been shown to improve brain function in subjects with cognitive dysfunction from long-term substance abuse (Schmitt 1984). Light therapy boxes, like those used to treat seasonal affective disorder, can also help. One of my patients with severe depression during the darker winter months has found that daily light therapy improved not only her mood but her fibrofog. If you also suffer from seasonal affective disorder or depression, it's certainly worth a try. The usual recommended dosage is twenty minutes first thing in the morning—it's easy to have it at the kitchen table and turn it on while you're eating breakfast or drinking your morning coffee. I like the Happylight line by Verilux.

You already learned about nutrients that can increase energy production, which have the added benefit of improving brain function. These powerhouse nutrients include alpha-lipoic acid, acetyl-L-carnitine, and CoQ10. They act as protectors of nerve cells and can improve memory and brain power (Packer 1997; Liu 2008; Kobayashi 2010; Orsucci 2011). Other nutrients that support nerves include activated B vitamins and omega-3 fatty acids (Suchy 2009). The good news is that these supplements can help both fibrofog *and* pain, but it can take time for the full benefits to become clear, so take them for at least three months before judging their effectiveness. One product that contains the right amounts of activated B vitamins, CoQ10, alpha-lipoic acid, and acetyl-L-carnitine is RevitalAge Nerve by Pure Encapsulations. If you take this along with fish oil for your omega-3s your brain will have all the nutrients it needs to fight the fog.

Key Brain Support Nutrients

Acetyl-L-carnitine 1,000 mg daily
Alpha-lipoic acid 400–600 mg daily
CoQ10 200–400 mg daily

Medications That Reduce Fibrofog

I have found several categories of medications useful for treating fibrofog. The first, memantine (Namenda), is commonly used to treat Alzheimer's, but it can help in cases of severe fibrofog. Steve, the veteran, noticed a huge change in his memory and ability to think on memantine. It also acts as a pain reducer, as you will learn more about in chapter 19, and Steve found it reduced his pain hypersensitivity as well. Other medications that can reduce fibrofog are antidepressants with a stimulating effect on the brain, in particular bupropion (Wellbutrin) and aripiprazole (Abilify).

Fibromyalgia patients have similar cognitive deficits to those seen in attention deficit disorder (Glass 2008). ADD is characterized by being easily distracted and having difficulty focusing, completing tasks, and processing information. You can see how this looks a lot like fibrofog, and many patients do benefit from medications that are used to treat ADD. Generally, it is treated with stimulants such as methylphenidate (Ritalin) or amphetamine/dextroamphetamine (Adderall). Unfortunately no studies have been done on using either for fibrofog, but adult patients with ADD and fibromyalgia who were treated with stimulants reported improvement in fog and fatigue (Young 2007). Some doctors don't like to prescribe stimulant medications to treat fibrofog, but may feel more comfortable if there is a confirmed diagnosis of ADD as well, and most of my fibromyalgia patients with severe fibrofog do meet the diagnostic criteria. If you suspect you have ADD, it's worth seeing a mental health practitioner for diagnosis and treatment.

Ways to Clear Fibrofog

- Exercise
- Cognitive training games
- Cranial electrotherapy stimulation
- Lightbox therapy
- Brain support nutrients
- NMDA-blocking medications
- Stimulant medications
- Activating antidepressants

To Do Yourself

- If your blood pressure runs below 100/60, increase salt intake and drink more water to keep blood pressure higher; the goal is around 120/80.
- If you are on blood pressure medications I highly encourage you to buy a monitor for home use so you can make sure you're not too low.

- Try www.verilux.com for light therapy boxes.
- Check out www.lumosity.com for brain-training games.
- Go to www.alphastim.com to learn about cranial electro-therapy stimulation (CES).

To Discuss with Your Health Care Provider

- Reducing or eliminating daytime doses of sedating medications, especially pregabalin (Lyrica), gabapentin (Neurontin), and/or muscle relaxants.
- Trying prescription stimulants, especially if you have fatigue and sleep apnea.
- If you're interested in ADD medications for fibrofog, a referral to be evaluated for ADD by a mental health practitioner.
- Trying stimulating antidepressants like Wellbutrin or Abilify.

CHAPTER 19

Reduce: Pain Hypersensitivity

*I feel like the Princess and the Pea, who can feel a
pea under forty mattresses.*
—FIBROMYALGIA PATIENT

A one-size-fits-all treatment approach to fibromyalgia pain
does not work. Within fibromyalgia there are actually three
separate types of pain, and each must be approached differently. The first is the vague, flulike aching caused by high levels
of inflammatory chemicals in the bloodstream. In the Rebalance section we covered ways to decrease inflammation and
reduce this type of pain. The second is muscle tenderness due
to tension and inflammation in the fascia, the connective tissue
that surrounds the muscle. The Repair section showed you how
to treat this with manual therapies, stretching, and trigger point
injections. The third is all-over sensitivity resulting from the
volume being turned way up in the nerves. This type of pain is
the trickiest to understand but has the most medication options, since it is where the pharmaceutical companies have focused most of their research.

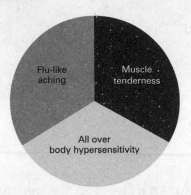

The three types of fibromyalgia pain.

Fortunately, lowering inflammation and treating fascial tightness will lessen your pain sensitivity. But for some patients that hypersensitivity will still remain problematic, and this chapter discusses other methods to combat it (medical marijuana and opiates are such complex issues that a separate chapter is devoted to each). Before we get into treatment, we need to understand more about what is causing a tap on your arm to feel like a punch.

Why Has Pain Gone Haywire in Fibromyalgia?

Pain is an electrical signal that travels from nerves up through the spinal cord to the brain. In fibromyalgia the signals from the pain-sensing nerves are amplified, which means even a small discomfort can be highly painful. Sensations not usually interpreted as pain, such as clothes resting on your skin, can be intensified to the point that they hurt as well.

Normally, as pain signals travel into the brain, they are processed and turned down. If pain signals are like a radio transmission, the spinal cord can turn the volume down and the brain can put in "earplugs" once the message has been received.

Imagine coming into a room where the radio is playing loudly and then turning up the dial and putting your ear right by the speaker. The sound would be nearly deafening. That is what is happening in fibromyalgia: the spinal cord and brain turn the pain volume *up* instead of turning it down as they should, in what is known as central sensitization (because the *central* nervous system has become more *sensitive* to pain) (Lee 2011; Murphy 2012; Cagnie 2014).

Why does pain sensitivity get ramped up in fibromyalgia? We have our old friend, the fight-or-flight nervous system, to thank. Constant fight-or-flight signaling acts as an irritant to the pain-sensing nerves and flares up hypersensitivity to pain. The other trigger is excessive pain signals from the muscles and other tissues that overwhelm the volume control system in the spinal cord and brain.

Turning Down the Volume on Pain

To reduce pain from nerve hypersensitivity we need to lower the volume on their signals along the pathway from the nerves to the spinal cord to the brain. The first step is to quiet the signals being sent into the spinal cord from all over the body. Think of pain hypersensitivity as a fire—the best way to put one out is to take away anything flammable. The fascia surrounding the muscles is the biggest generator of pain signals in fibromyalgia, which is why treatments directed at painful and tight fascial areas, as you learned in chapter 12, are so important. Many people with fibromyalgia have other sources of pain that are feeding the hypersensitivity fire, such as joint pain from arthritis or nerve pain from neuropathy (see chapter 22 for more on treating common causes of pain).

The primary pain signals streaming into the spinal cord are coming from irritated nerve endings in the muscle and surrounding fascia. To quiet them we need to reduce muscle inflammation, block fight-or-flight nerves, and protect pain-sensing nerves from damage. The hypersensitized spinal cord turns up the volume on pain in response to inflammation and high levels of pain-enhancing chemicals, so anything to curb those chemicals and reduce inflammation in the spinal cord helps normalize pain volume. Finally, treatments that increase the brain's ability to filter out more of the pain "noise" will turn down the dial as well.

Where Pain Treatments Block Signals

Pain-Sensing Nerves in Muscle
- Beta-blockers
- Topical NSAIDs
- Compounded pain cream
- Supplements to protect nerves

Spinal Cord
- Anticonvulsants
- Avoiding dietary excitotoxins
- NMDA receptor blockers
- Lidocaine/mexiletine
- Low-dose naltrexone

Brain
- Serotonin-norepinephrine reuptake inhibitors (SNRIs)
- Dopamine medications
- Cranial electrotherapy stimulation
- Changing thought patterns

Muscle: Calming Fight-or-Flight Nerves

The chronic stress response in fibromyalgia means that the fight-or-flight nerves are continually active, directing the pain-sensing nerves to send louder signals from the muscles in particular. We can reduce discomfort by reducing the activity of those nerves so they cause less irritation to the pain sensors. Several types of medications can help. The most common are the beta-blockers, usually used as treatment for high blood pressure, which inhibit the action of signaling chemicals used by the fight-or-flight nerves. Some beta-blocker medications, including atenolol and metoprolol, primarily work on the heart, whereas others block fight-or-flight nerves in both the heart and in muscles; those are the ones we use in fibromyalgia. Pindolol and propranolol can both reduce fibromyalgia pain (Wood 2005; Light 2009). Linda, my patient with Lyme disease and fibromyalgia, had a significant abatement in pain once she started pindolol.

Beta-blockers interfere with melatonin production in the brain (Stoschitzky 1999). Melatonin is an important trigger for sleep, so if you take beta-blockers be sure to supplement with melatonin at bedtime. They can also lower your blood pressure or heart rate, so if you have low blood pressure or a slow heart rate you may not be able to tolerate them. I usually prescribe minimal doses and work up gradually, which improves tolerance. If you are on another medication for high blood pressure, talk to your doctor about trying pindolol or propranolol instead.

Another way to lessen fight-or-flight signals in the muscle is through the topical application of alpha-blockers, the most common of which is clonidine. I often prescribe a compounded pain cream for fibromyalgia that includes clonidine, and I have found it very effective for local pain relief (Campbell 2012).

(See the compounded medication section below and on the following page for more details.)

Muscle: Reducing Inflammation

Inflammation in the muscles and fascia also irritates the pain-sensing nerves. Nonsteroidal anti-inflammatory medications (NSAIDs) taken orally are not very effective for fibromyalgia pain, but when applied to the skin over the muscle they seep into tissue and can be highly effective (Yunus 1989). NSAIDs show up at a concentration four to seven times greater in muscular tissue after topical versus oral administration (Tegeder 1999; Dominkus 1996). Additionally, while oral NSAIDs can irritate the stomach lining and have other side effects, very little of the topical versions reach the bloodstream, so they carry fewer risks (Heyneman 2000). Topical NSAIDs have been used for many years in Europe, and are often available over the counter there. Three prescription formulations are available in the United States. Although the FDA approves their use only for osteoarthritis-related knee and hand pain, they can be effective on any localized area of muscle or fascial discomfort (Hsieh 2010; Argoff 2002).

Prescription Topical NSAIDs

Flector patch (diclofenac topical patch)
Voltaren gel (diclofenac 1 percent gel)
Pennsaid (diclofenac topical solution 1.5 percent)

NSAIDs can also be added to specially compounded creams that contain several other medications to lower pain signals.

Compounding pharmacies customize combinations of prescription medications that are mixed together into a cream or gel and applied topically. The most effective ones contain an NSAID in addition to a numbing medication, clonidine to block fight-or-flight nerve signals, and gabapentin and ketamine to reduce painful nerve signals (Lynch 2005; Uzaraga 2012; Finch 2009).

Common Ingredients in a Topical Compounded Fibromyalgia Pain Cream

lidocaine or tetracaine—numbing agent
diclofenac or ketoprofen—NSAID
clonidine—fight-or-flight nerve blocker
gabapentin—nerve pain blocker
ketamine—nerve pain blocker and opiate receptor
   stimulator

Muscle: Protecting Pain-Sensing Nerves

Pain-sensing nerves that are subjected to excess inflammation and irritating fight-or-flight nerve signals can actually suffer damage, causing even more pain. In fibromyalgia this is exacerbated by the fact that chronic muscle tension causes the muscle cells to burn through their energy stores quickly, which leads to an inflammatory cycle. Recent studies show that nearly half of the fibromyalgia subjects showed evidence of nerve damage, or neuropathy, similar to that seen in diabetes (Üçeyler June 2013; Oaklander 2013). Nerve damage results in pain, numbness and tingling, and, in more severe cases, loss of sensation.

It is vital to protect nerves from damage caused by inflammation. We can do this by supplementing with nutrients to support the mitochondria, the "furnaces" that produce energy for muscle cells. You learned about how to bolster mitochondrial function with alpha-lipoic acid, CoQ10, and acetyl-L-carnitine in the Repair chapters. Alpha-lipoic acid is a powerful antioxidant that has also been shown to help reduce nerve damage and improve nerve pain (Ametov 2003; Ziegler 2004, 2006).

Spinal Cord: Medications to Lower Pain-Enhancing Chemicals

Let's shift focus from blocking pain signals in the muscles to lowering their magnification as they pass up the spinal cord. One way to do that is by reducing the amount of pain-enhancing chemicals in the spinal cord with medications like pregabalin (Lyrica) and gabapentin (Neurontin). Both have been found to reduce pain in fibromyalgia (Üçeyler Oct 2013; Arnold 2007). Only pregabalin is FDA-approved for that use, but gabapentin, an older and much cheaper medication, has a similar impact. Both can cause side effects, including sedation, weight gain, water retention, and dizziness. In clinical trials, 19 to 33 percent of patients on pregabalin stopped treatment due to its side effects (Prescrire Int. 2009). I often prescribe these medications just at bedtime, or at a lower dose during the day and a higher one at bedtime to limit their sedating side effects. As you learned in chapter 9, both increase the amount of deep sleep, so taking them at night is optimal to improve sleep quality. Although only pregabalin and gabapentin have been studied for fibromyalgia, another similar medication, topiramate (Topamax), can also be beneficial (Kararizou 2013).

FAQ: What if pregabalin or gabapentin is helping my pain but I am having side effects?

Side effects can be reduced by keeping doses low, so I will often try slowly lowering the dosage to its minimum effective dose. If you are having side effects with one of these medications it's also worth trying a switch to the other. People may have side effects with one but not the other. If the medications are working but are causing water retention, I prescribe a low-dose diuretic (water pill) as well.

It is important to avoid medications that can increase pain-enhancing chemicals in the spinal cord, in particular a category commonly prescribed for high blood pressure. ACE inhibitors lower blood pressure by blocking the production of chemicals that constrict blood vessels—the blood vessel dilates and blood pressure goes down. But they also inhibit the breakdown of pain-enhancing chemicals in the spinal cord (de Mos 2009). I usually switch my patients on ACE inhibitors over to similar medications called ARBs that do not have that particular negative effect.

ACE Inhibitors (Fibromyalgia Pain Elevators)
lisinopril (Zestril, Prinivil)
captopril (Capoten)
enalapril (Vasotec)
ramipril (Altace)
quinapril (Accupril)
benazepril (Lotensin)

trandolapril (Mavik)

perindopril (Aceon)

moexipril (Univasc)

fosinopril (Monopril)

ARBs (Fibromyalgia Pain Neutral)

candesartan (Atacand)

eprosartan (Teveten)

irbesartan (Avapro)

telmisartan (Micardis)

valsartan (Diovan)

losartan (Cozaar)

olmesartan (Benicar) .

You should also be aware that when high daily doses of opiate pain meds are used long term, they provoke the spinal cord cells to make more pain-enhancing chemicals and can actually increase pain (Watkins 2007). This is called opiate-induced hyperalgesia, which I describe how to avoid in chapter 20.

Spinal Cord: Dietary Changes to Lower Pain-Enhancing Chemicals

Amazingly, the foods we eat can also affect the levels of pain-enhancing chemicals in our spinal cord. Glutamate is one of the most potent pain enhancers and is also found in our diet, most commonly in the form of monosodium glutamate (MSG) as a flavor enhancer and food preservative. The artificial sweetener known as aspartame is converted in the body to aspartate, which is another bad guy for pain. Aspartate and glutamate are known as dietary excitotoxins, which means they are in what we eat and are known to be irritating to the brain and spinal cord. They can also worsen fibromyalgia pain, so I recommend completely avoiding MSG and aspartame (Smith 2001).

In one study, 80 percent of subjects who did not consume any aspartame or MSG for four weeks recorded a significant reduction in symptoms. And when given a blinded MSG challenge (in which they were given either MSG or a placebo), those who received MSG noted a significant return of their symptoms (Holton 2012). I have had several patients whose pain levels dropped after they stopped drinking diet soda, including Pam, who you may remember was a self-described "Diet Coke addict." I can always tell when I have accidentally eaten something that contains MSG. Within a few hours I feel a weird itchy burning sensation all over my body and any existing mild pain becomes severe pain. It is such an unpleasant experience that I work really hard to avoid MSG!

FAQ: Do all artificial sweeteners flare up fibromyalgia pain?

In addition to aspartame, almost all artificial sweeteners, including sucralose (Splenda) and saccharin (Sweet'N Low), can hike up fibromyalgia pain. Corn syrup can be inflammatory as well, so try to consume only cane or beet sugar. Believe it or not, it is better to just eat real sugar! The best non-sugar sweetener is stevia, which is made from the leaves of a plant and is not a dietary excitotoxin.

Dietary Sources of Pain-Enhancing Chemicals to Avoid

monosodium glutamate (MSG)
monopotassium glutamate
glutamate
hydrolyzed protein
textured protein
sodium caseinate
calcium caseinate
autolyzed yeast
yeast extract
gelatin
aspartame
saccharin
sucralose

Spinal Cord: Block the Action of Pain-Enhancing Chemicals

Along with lowering the load of pain-enhancing chemicals, we can also use medications to block their activity. Blocking glutamate from binding to the NMDA receptor reduces pain signal transmission. Medications that do just that, called NMDA receptor blockers, have been approved to treat Alzheimer's dementia and have been shown to reduce discomfort in other conditions characterized by hyperactive pain signals (Recla 2009; Kleinböhl 2006; Amin 2003). They include memantine (Namenda) and amantadine (Symmetrel). One study found that memantine reduced pain in fibromyalgia over a period of six months, and subjects also reported improved cognitive functioning, which makes sense since the original purpose of the drug was to recover brain function in dementia (Olivan-Blázquez 2014). Steve, the veteran you met in the treatment overview, found memantine helpful for his pain and fibrofog.

Quite a few patients of mine have registered significant pain reduction on memantine. It is generally very well tolerated as long as the dosage starts low and increases slowly. It is currently quite expensive and is only FDA-approved to treat dementia, so using it for fibromyalgia is considered off-label and not covered by many insurance plans. However, if further studies show benefit for fibromyalgia, it may gain approval. Amantadine is a weaker NMDA blocker and therefore not as effective, but it is much cheaper so still a good option.

FAQ: What does using a medication "off-label" mean?

"Off-label" means using a medication for a condition that it was not FDA-approved to treat. When the Food and Drug Administration (FDA) approves the sale of a pharmaceutical drug in the United States, it only does so for those diseases on which there is research data to support the usage. For example, diabetes medications are approved only for use in diabetes. Many medications have research supporting their prescription for other conditions, but the companies making them may choose not to pursue official approval since it is such an expensive process. Sometimes health insurance companies refuse to pay for medications prescribed off-label, even though this includes a quarter of all prescriptions written in the United States (Radley 2006). For example, pregabalin (Lyrica) is FDA-approved for fibromyalgia, but the very similar and commonly prescribed gabapentin is not.

Spinal Cord: Numbing the Spinal Cord Pain Signals

We can also block spinal cord pain signals by numbing them. Lidocaine is a common local anesthetic (numbing) agent that is used in surgery and dental procedures. When given intravenously it lowers pain signals in the spinal cord and can temporarily reduce fibromyalgia pain. A few of my patients have found that lidocaine infusions diminish their pain for about a week. One study found that this medicine reduced pain in fibromyalgia more than IV morphine, and others have confirmed significant, but temporary, results (Sörensen 1995; McCleane 2000; Schafranski 2009). The major drawback is its side effects, which can include dangerously slow or fast heart rates (Raphael 2003). Safety concerns, coupled with only short-term benefits, have limited its use in fibromyalgia. However, a related oral medication called mexiletine (Mexitil) may have longer-lasting pain relief and is safer—although not risk-free.

Mexiletine is usually used to treat abnormal heart rhythms, but can also be used off-label for pain. Nine studies have found mexiletine helpful for pain from nerve damage (Tremont-Lukats 2005). No published research has yet been done on mexiletine and fibromyalgia, but a pain management colleague of mine has found it effective for a few of his fibromyalgia patients. He prescribes it only for people who respond well to a monitored IV lidocaine "challenge" in the clinic to make sure they can tolerate it. Mexiletene can also cause dangerously irregular heartbeats in people with heart problems, so many doctors don't feel comfortable prescribing it. However, the safety concerns may be overstated. One analysis of thirty studies on IV lidocaine and oral mexiletine concluded that "systemic local anesthetics were safe, with no deaths or life-threatening toxicities" (Challapalli 2005). Still, I recommend you work with a pain specialist familiar with the potential risks if you choose to pursue this type of treatment.

Spinal Cord: Reduce Inflammation

Just as inflammation irritates the pain-sensing nerves, it also irritates the pain-transmitting cells in the spinal cord. By reducing inflammation in the spinal cord we lower the volume of pain transmitted to the brain. Curcumin, the active anti-inflammatory in the spice turmeric, can calm this type of irritation (Choi 2011). See chapter 14 for more information on this supplement.

The most effective way to reduce spinal cord inflammation is with a medication called low-dose naltrexone (LDN). Naltrexone is a medication used to treat addiction because it blocks opiate receptors. It also acts as anti-inflammatory in the spinal cord. Stanford University researchers found in two separate studies that LDN reduced fibromyalgia pain by as much as 30 percent (Younger 2013, 2014). Side effects were infrequent and were usually headache, vivid dreams, insomnia, or anxiety. In my experience, side effects are minimal when dosage is increased slowly, and it can take twenty-eight days to reach peak effectiveness. If it causes insomnia, LDN can be taken in the morning.

I have had several patients improve with low-dose naltrexone, but there are two challenges to prescribing it. First, it has to be specially made by a compounding pharmacy, and many doctors are not used to writing compounded prescriptions. Second, LDN does not mix well with opiate pain medications. Since it is an opiate blocker, it can counteract the pain relief of opiates.

FAQ: Can I take opiate pain medications while on LDN?

Since naltrexone is an opiate blocker, it can render opiate pain medications ineffective and even trigger withdrawal (diarrhea, sweating, and nausea) for those on daily opiates. I avoid using LDN with patients who take daily long-acting opiate medications (fentanyl patch, MS Contin, methadone, OxyContin, Butrans patch, or Tramadol ER). I advise patients on occasional short-acting pain meds to take them at least six hours apart from LDN.

Brain: Increase Ability to Filter Out Pain Signals

Moving up from the spinal cord, there are several ways we can help the brain to filter out more of the pain "noise." Medications that increase serotonin, norepinephrine, and dopamine have been shown to reduce fibromyalgia pain. A non-medication approach is cranial electrotherapy stimulation (CES), which can help the brain filter out pain signals. Subjects using CES had more reduction in pain than those using fake devices. Additionally, brain imaging found that individuals using a CES device had lower activity in the pain-processing regions of the brain compared to those using a fake one (Taylor 2013).

Medications that improve the brain's pain filters include serotonin-norepinephrine reuptake inhibitor (SNRI) antidepressants, which increase brain serotonin and norepinephrine levels: duloxetine (Cymbalta), milnacipran (Savella), and venlafaxine (Effexor). SNRIs are quite effective at reducing pain hypersensitivity, and both duloxetine and milnacipran are FDA-approved for fibromyalgia (Clauw 2008). Some of my patients report up to a 40 percent reduction in their pain levels, and since SNRIs also boost mood they are an especially good choice if you also have depression. They are generally well tolerated, but the most common side effects are nausea, excess sweating, and increased heart rate. If they are working for pain but the side effect of sweating is troublesome, I will add a medication called prazosin to reduce sweating.

The other medications that help the brain to filter more pain signals are those that increase dopamine, commonly prescribed for restless legs syndrome: ropinirole (Requip), pramipexole (Mirapex), and carbidopa/levodopa (Sinemet). A study on pramipexole found improvement in pain, fatigue, and functioning in fibromyalgia, but side effects included weight loss, nausea, and anxiety (Holman 2005). The most concerning side effect is the sudden onset of an impulse control disorder, like gambling, excessive shopping, or hypersexuality. One of my patients began compulsively collecting rocks, and another couldn't stop ordering from TV shopping programs. These side effects limit the usefulness of these medications in fibromyalgia, but they are worth considering if you also have restless legs syndrome.

Brain: Using Conscious Thought to Change Pain Experience

Research shows that how we think about pain actually affects how much attention our brain pays to its signals. Brain imaging shows that pain catastrophizing (characterizing pain as "unbearable," "horrible," or "awful") is significantly associated with increased activity in the areas related to pain (Gracely 2004). This is one area where we can put our brain to work for us!

There are many methods we can employ to change how we think about pain, and developing those skills to help change our internal dialogue can be very constructive. One simple way is by using positive affirmations. It feels ridiculous at first, but thinking or saying out loud things like "this flare-up will pass quickly" or "I am happy despite this pain" can be truly effective. In one study, patients were simply given a script to read aloud in front of others in weekly meetings. Those who read aloud "I am able to cope well with pain" reported lesser symptoms over time than those who said, "I am not able to cope with pain" (Gilliam 2013).

Changing how you think about pain can turn it from a scream to a whisper. A pain psychologist or counselor can help you recognize and alter unhealthy thought patterns. Cognitive-behavioral therapy (CBT) is particularly beneficial in improving negative ways of thinking like overgeneralizing, magnifying negatives, minimizing positives, and catastrophizing. It has also been shown to help reduce pain and improve quality of life for sufferers of various chronic pain conditions (Hoffman 2007). I particularly like the Mastering Pain Method, which is the brainchild of a pain psychologist who herself suffers from chronic pain. Her self-guided program online has been really helpful for quite a few of my patients.

I've just presented you with a lot of options, and as always, don't feel you have to try all of them. Talk with your HCP to determine which ones might be best for you. Any treatment that lowers pain signals along their path from nerves to the spinal cord and onto the brain will lessen hypersensitivity—so you won't feel a pea under forty mattresses anymore.

To Do Yourself

- Avoid dietary excitotoxins (MSG and artificial sweeteners).
- Consider cranial electrotherapy stimulation (CES); you can find more information in chapter 7.

- Work on modifying your internal dialogue about pain to avoid catastrophizing. Check out www .masteringpainmethod.com, *Master Your Pain* by Jill Fancher, and *Managing Pain Before It Manages You* by Margaret Caudill.

To Discuss with Your Health Care Provider

- If you are currently taking an ACE inhibitor for high blood pressure, ask about changing to an ARB.
- Consider taking an SNRI, especially if you also have depression.
- Consider trying a dopamine agonist, especially if you also have RLS.
- Consider low-dose naltrexone if you don't take daily opiates (talk to a naturopath or holistic provider).
- If you're interested in mexiletine, request a referral to a pain specialist.
- Consider taking an anticonvulsant.
- Try NMDA blockers, especially if you also have severe fibrofog.

CHAPTER 20

Reduce: Opiates for Pain Relief

The use of opiate-based pain medications (also called opioids) for fibromyalgia is very controversial—in fact, all current medical guidelines advise against their use. It can be confusing and frustrating for patients who wonder why their doctors are so hesitant to prescribe them this form of pain relief. It boils down to this: in published studies, opioids haven't been shown to work very well. One medical journal wrote that "opioid use for the management of pain in fibromyalgia is strongly discouraged and is not recommended by any current practice guideline" (Fitzcharles 2011). But because doctors don't have much else to offer their fibromyalgia patients, many end up reluctantly prescribing them opiates (Berger 2010).

The guidelines advising doctors to not prescribe opiates are derived from a few small studies showing they were ineffective for fibromyalgia pain. Keep in mind that there are no large studies that have examined this issue, so doctors are making decisions without much information. Most of what I have learned about managing fibromyalgia pain is from my extensive experience treating patients; I have learned both how to prescribe opiates correctly and what to avoid. Most doctors do not have this clinical background, so instead must rely on recommendations from the little research out there.

Opioids have a medicinal effect on humans because we already have receptors in our brain and body for similar chemicals that our body naturally makes called endorphins. These chemicals block pain signals and regulate inflammation. Opiate-based medications activate these same pain-blocking receptors and effectively relieve acute or short-term pain, but when used chronically they can sometimes have the opposite effect and actually make pain *worse*. But they are useful tools if applied in the right way. This chapter reviews the pros and cons, and what experience has taught me about how best to utilize them for fibromyalgia.

Studies on Opiates for Fibromyalgia Pain

We don't have much data on using opiates to manage fibromyalgia pain, but what we do have does not support their use. In a multidisciplinary pain clinic, fibromyalgia patients who were prescribed opiates had worse symptoms over time compared to the group who were not (Fitzcharles 2013).

In two large studies, the weak opiate tramadol has been shown to be effective for fibromyalgia pain. Likely much of the benefit here comes not from its opiate activity but instead its effect on other chemicals in the brain that suppress pain signals (Bennett 2003; Russell 2000). The few studies that have been done on stronger opiates show that they don't work that well. For example, a one-time dosage of IV morphine did not result in any noticeable pain improvement for thirty-one patients (Sörensen 1995). Another study followed forty-three people for four years as they received opiate therapy; their overall pain scores went down a little (average pain improved from a 7.8 to a 7), but measures of function and mood got worse (Kemple 2003).

Since no large randomized controlled trials have been done, the recommendations against opiate use are based on data from less than a hundred subjects! Most of the medical guidelines take into consideration some larger studies that show that opiates are ineffective for other chronic pain conditions like low back pain and peripheral neuropathy, but we should use caution in extrapolating this data to fibromyalgia—it is a distinct disease that responds to different treatments.

Opiate-Based Pain Medications

morphine
morphine sustained release (MS Contin)
codeine
hydrocodone/acetaminophen (Vicodin, Norco, Lortab)
oxycodone
oxycodone/acetaminophen (Percocet)
oxycodone extended release (OxyContin)
methadone
fentanyl patch
hydromorphone (Dilaudid)
buprenorphine (Suboxone, Butrans patch)
tramadol (Ultram, Ryzolt)
tapentadol (Nucynta, Nucynta ER)

Problems Caused by Long-Term Opiate Use

Long-term daily use of opiate-based pain medications causes several problems. The body develops a tolerance, so they lose effectiveness over time. You can also develop dependence on opiates, so if they are stopped suddenly you may experience unpleasant withdrawal symptoms, including increased pain, anxiety, nausea, vomiting, sweating, and diarrhea. Long-term use also causes hormonal changes in the body, in particular lowering testosterone levels and impairing the ability of the adrenal glands to make steroid hormones. Because opiates can cause euphoria or a high, there is also a risk of misuse and abuse (Benyamin 2008).

But the biggest problem is that over time they can actually *increase* pain. When taken chronically, they can lead to opiate-induced hyperalgesia, meaning increased pain caused by the medication itself. The condition is characterized by a paradoxical response in which pain becomes worse the higher the dosage. One study of chronic pain patients on high-dose opioids found that twenty-one out of twenty-three reported a significant decrease in pain after stopping the medicine (Baron 2006).

How could medications to reduce pain have such a markedly opposite effect? Well, we know that over time long-term high-dose opioids increase pain-enhancing chemicals in the spinal cord. In addition, they activate spinal glial cells, which increase sensitivity to pain signals. Essentially, the spinal cord starts turning up the volume on pain signals. Since in fibromyalgia the body is already doing that, you can see how opiates might make a bad situation even worse (Lee 2011).

FAQ: What is considered a high dose of opiates?

Doctors use "morphine equivalents" to compare different opiates, and any daily dosage that is equivalent to 120 mg of morphine or more is considered high. You can reference online calculators that convert dosages of different opioids to their morphine equivalents, or ask your HCP. Remember to never make any dosage changes without talking to your provider first.

Daily Opiate Amount Considered High Dose

fentanyl 50 mcg patch

morphine 120 mg

oxycodone 80 mg

hydrocodone 100 mg

methadone 30 mg

hydromorphone 25 mg

oxymorphone 40 mg

Using Opiates to Best Effect in Fibromyalgia

Even with our knowledge that opioids are imperfect tools for long-term pain management, until we have more effective symptomatic treatments they can still play an important role. As with any tool, we need to utilize them in the right way. I have found that small amounts of low-dose opiates used occasionally during pain flares can be helpful without triggering hyperalgesia. I try to avoid regular doses of opioids such as oxycodone and hydrocodone, as they can rapidly create tolerance and increase pain over time, but as long as they are used intermittently, not every day, that's less of a concern. A good rule of thumb is to limit "as needed" dosing to ten days a month, or less than 30 percent of the time, which seems to hinder the development of negative side effects. For the most part, my patients do better overall when not taking opiates daily, but if a more frequent prescription is necessary, I try to choose one that has a lower chance of causing opiate-induced hyperalgesia: tramadol, tapentadol, buprenorphine, or low-dose methadone. And remember that opiates have a negative impact on sleep quality, so avoid taking them within four hours of bedtime (Shaw 2005).

Using Opiates Wisely for Fibromyalgia Pain

- Avoid high-dose opiates.
- Keep as-needed use to less than 30 percent of days.
- For daily usage take one that causes less hyperalgesia.
- Keep opiates away from bedtime to limit sleep interference.

The only opiate that studies have shown to be effective for fibromyalgia is tramadol—although to be fair, no others have specifically been studied for the condition. As you've already learned, tramadol is a unique medication that has opiate activity but also increases serotonin and norepinephrine in the brain. These neurotransmitters boost the brain's ability to filter out pain signals, and enable tramadol to act as a mild antidepressant. Many patients find that it improves both mood and pain. It also has a lower abuse potential than other opiates, and until 2014 was not treated as a controlled substance in the United States. Note that it can be dangerous to combine with medications that also increase serotonin levels, like antidepressants. Serotonin syndrome, a relatively rare condition of excess serotonin in the brain, can be life-threatening, with a rapid onset of symptoms including confusion, fast heart rate, hallucinations, increased body temperature, and even seizures. This risk unfortunately limits the use of tramadol in patients who are already taking antidepressants. A similar newer medication is tapentadol, although this has not been specifically studied for fibromyalgia pain. It has a lower risk of serotonin syndrome, as it does not increase levels of serotonin to the same degree.

FAQ: How do I avoid serotonin syndrome?

Serotonin syndrome develops most often when different types of drugs that increase serotonin levels (opiate-based pain medications, antidepressants, and migraine medications) are combined. To avoid it, make sure you ask your pharmacist or HCP before filling a new prescription or starting a new supplement. If you suspect you might have serotonin syndrome after starting a new drug or increasing a dose, seek emergency treatment immediately. Serotonin syndrome is extremely rare, but it is important to be aware of it because early medical intervention can save your life!

Buprenorphine is a unique opioid that only partly activates the opiate receptor. Think of buprenorphine as someone standing on the threshold of an open door, with one foot in the room and one in the hallway. This makes it less likely to cause tolerance, so doses can remain low and still be effective. It also is less likely to cause the increased pain associated with long-term opiate use and thus is referred to as an "antihyperalgesic" (Koppert 2005). Buprenorphine is not well absorbed in the stomach, so it comes in a transdermal patch (Butrans) and sublingual tablets. For some patients, the patch, which is changed only once a week, is very helpful for pain. It can be irritating to the skin, though, so if this is a problem try pretreating the area with topical hydrocortisone cream the day before adhering a patch.

Methadone has the special property of blocking the NMDA receptor, in addition to activating opiate receptors. You might recall from the last chapter that medications that block the

NMDA receptor help turn down the pain volume in the spinal cord. It is also less likely to cause tolerance or escalate pain levels over time (Salpeter 2013; Lee 2011). However, methadone can be tricky, because although its pain-relieving effects only last about eight hours, it sticks around in the body for three to five days. Increasing your dose needs to be done very slowly so that levels can build up gradually in the body. Methadone is also associated with triggering abnormal heartbeats in people with certain heart conditions, so I always check a screening EKG before I prescribe it, and I keep doses low, under 30 mg daily.

FAQ: Isn't methadone prescribed to drug addicts?

Methadone is used as "medication-assisted treatment" to treat opioid and heroin addiction. It is dosed very differently and prescribed by doctors who are addiction specialists. However, it is also commonly used as a pain medication. If you take methadone for pain it does not mean you are a drug addict!

Patients taking opiates often worry that they will become addicted. The term "addiction" is often used incorrectly to mean "dependence," but there is a very important distinction between the two. Dependence simply means that your body becomes used to a medicine to the point that if you stop it suddenly you will experience withdrawal. It can happen with many different types of medications, not just opiates. If you take opiate medications daily, your body will become dependent on them, and if you quit suddenly you may have symptoms such as nausea, diarrhea, anxiety, sweating, and muscle aches (known colloquially as the "opiate flu"). Everyone who takes opiates daily becomes dependent on them, but addiction happens to only a small percentage.

Addiction, on the other hand, means misusing a substance to get high or to change one's mood, not for pain relief. Signs include compulsive use of the medication, lying about use, and not being able to control use, even when it may be causing damage to a person's life, job, or family. People with a past history of substance abuse are more likely to develop addiction problems with opiates.

Another Complicating Factor

In a new twist, we are just now learning that people metabolize opiates differently. Any medication that you take has to be processed into a form that your body can eliminate. This is primarily done in the liver by a group of enzymes called cytochrome P450. We all have the same enzymes, but they vary in how effectively they are able to clear medications out of our system. Some people have weak enzymes and will metabolize certain drugs slowly; they need much lower doses. Others have enzymes that metabolize medications very quickly, and require higher doses. In particular, there are several opiates that vary in how well they are processed by the body, including codeine, oxycodone, and tramadol. This is a very new area of medicine, but I predict in the future we will start testing patients' ability to metabolize a medication before we prescribe it. There are already some genetic tests that can be done with blood or oral swabs to learn your overall makeup of these enzymes, so if interested, talk with your HCP.

So Should I Use Opiates for Fibromyalgia Pain or Not?

Until we have better options, it is reasonable to use opiates as long as they are taken in such a way that they do not make fibromyalgia pain worse. The best way to do this is by avoiding daily use, reserving them for only the most severe episodes. By limiting as-needed dosing to ten days a month or fewer, you are unlikely to develop tolerance or heightened pain from hyperalgesia. If you do take daily opiate-based pain medications, remember that tramadol, tapentadol, buprenorphine, and low-dose methadone are the least likely to cause increased pain levels. Never make any changes to your doses or schedule of medications without talking first with your HCP.

In the next chapter you will learn about medical marijuana, an option that is becoming available to more and more patients. Marijuana may prove to be a much better treatment than opiates for fibromyalgia because it can decrease your central sensitivity to pain.

To Do Yourself

- Start tracking your pain levels daily. Bring this information to your HCP to help her make treatment decisions. It can also help you see if opiates are reducing or increasing your pain.
- Rate pain on a scale of 0 to 10, with 0 being no pain and 10 being the worst pain imaginable. Record one number as your pain score for each day on a calendar or in a notebook.
- Use an app designed to track pain levels. A popular one is www.chronicpainapp.com.

To Discuss with Your Health Care Provider

- Bring records of your daily pain tracking scores to your appointment.
- Ask if you are taking what is considered a high daily dosage of opiates (equivalent to 120 mg of morphine or more).
- Inquire about genetic testing for variations in drug-metabolizing enzymes.

CHAPTER 21

Reduce: Medical Marijuana for Pain Relief

At least once a day, a patient asks me if marijuana might help with their symptoms. The short answer is yes, but we don't have very many studies to back that up. Many of my patients do report that it reduces their pain and improves sleep, and several have been able to come off high doses of opiates completely and use only marijuana for pain management. One reported that it decreased her pain level from an 8 to a 3 on a 10-point scale. In contrast, prescription Cymbalta only brought her from an 8 to a 6, and opiates didn't help at all.

Despite a lack of official research, word of mouth among fibromyalgia sufferers means that marijuana is used frequently for symptom management. One Canadian study found that of almost five hundred fibromyalgia patients referred to a pain center, 13 percent were using medical marijuana (Ste-Marie 2012). Many doctors feel uncomfortable recommending its use, mostly because of contradictions between state and federal policy in the United States, leaving patients in the unenviable (but all too familiar) position of having to figure it out on their own.

Although it is often called marijuana, the preferred term for medical usage is cannabis. Cannabis is now legal for medical use in nearly half of U.S. states but is still classified as illegal by the federal government, giving it only a semilegal status. Its medicinal use remains controversial because it is classified under federal law as a drug with a "high potential for abuse" and "no currently accepted medical use." This is in direct contradiction to those states that have legalized marijuana for medical purposes, and the disconnect puts physicians in a legal gray zone that makes many hesitant to recommend its use. For this reason, there are very few doctors knowledgeable about its use, especially for fibromyalgia. I practice medicine in Oregon, a state that has a well-established medical marijuana program, with over sixty thousand patients currently registered. This area of the law is changing fast; resources to find updated information about your state are listed at the end of the chapter.

Does Marijuana Reduce Fibromyalgia Symptoms?

In 2000 B.C. the Chinese emperor Shen-Nung described marijuana's ability to diminish pain and inflammation and noted that it "undoes rheumatism" (an antiquated term for fibromyalgia) (Mack 2000). More recently, a study of twenty-eight fibromyalgia patients reported that two hours after use of cannabis they had a significant reduction of pain and stiffness, enhancement of relaxation, and an increased sense of well-being (Fiz 2011). Marijuana has also been studied and found effective for other painful conditions such as nerve damage from diabetes, multiple sclerosis, and rheumatoid arthritis (Rog 2005; Ware Oct 2010; Wade 2003).

Dronabinol (Marinol), a prescription synthetic tetrahydrocannabinol (THC), the main active ingredient in marijuana, reduced fibromyalgia pain but caused a lot of side effects in one small study (Schley 2006). In fact, more than half of the subjects withdrew due to side effects including dry mouth, dizziness, poor balance, and nausea. Another similar prescription medication called nabilone (Cesamet) was also effective for pain relief but again had a high rate of side effects (Skrabek

2008). I have found that some of my patients tolerate these fairly well, and for one dronabinol was so effective that it enabled him to return to work after several years on disability. Unfortunately, they are both expensive and often not covered by insurance for fibromyalgia.

Marijuana has demonstrated positive effects on sleep by increasing the amount of time spent in deep sleep. Fibromyalgia subjects reported improved quality of sleep and feeling more rested in the morning while on nabilone, but again reported side effects (Ware Feb 2010).

FAQ: Why does prescription THC have so many side effects?

Marijuana plants contain many other compounds in addition to THC, some of which are thought to limit its less pleasant side effects. The combination of active ingredients has an "entourage effect" that explains the better results with marijuana than with THC medications alone. In particular, an active ingredient called cannabidiol (CBD) has calming effects that counteract some of the undesirable ones like anxiety or feeling stoned or high. In Canada and Europe, a cannabis-based medical extract is approved for use as an oral spray (Sativex). It is entirely derived from a specially grown plant with extensive quality control and balanced amounts of THC and CBD, and it has been shown to significantly lessen pain and improve sleep for rheumatoid arthritis, with few side effects (Blake 2006). This product is currently undergoing clinical trials in the United States and it is hoped that it will be available within the next few years.

The Science of Marijuana

Marijuana (cannabis) has a medicinal effect on humans because we already have receptors in our brain and bodies for similar chemicals that our body naturally makes. Endocannabinoids are similar to our endorphins, which are morphine-like chemicals that block pain signals and regulate inflammation. Endocannabinoid levels in the body, which increase in response to exercise, have strong anti-inflammatory actions (Sparling 2003; Dietrich 2004).

In addition to THC, marijuana contains at least eighty other cannabinoids—which are defined as any chemical that activates the cannabinoid receptors in the body. Many cannabinoids have the effect of "speeding up the resolution of inflammation" (Burstein 2009). The most common non-psychoactive cannabinoid in marijuana is cannabidiol (CBD), which has very strong anti-inflammatory properties. Studies on CBD have shown that it reduces joint inflammation in mouse arthritis and suppresses the body's release of inflammatory chemicals (Sumariwalla 2004; Costa 2007).

There are two types of cannabinoid receptors in the body. Cannabinoid receptor type 1 (CB1) is found in the brain and nerves, and cannabinoid receptor type 2 (CB2) on immune cells. THC primarily activates CB1 receptors in the brain, where it blocks pain signals and causes the psychotropic effect of feeling high. Cannabinoids that stimulate CB2 receptors on immune cells block the release of painful inflammatory chemicals and reduce the release of substance P, a pain signal transmitter (Manzanares 2006).

Cannabinoids and Fibromyalgia

Fibromyalgia is characterized by hyperreactivity to pain in the brain and spinal cord called central sensitization, which has been linked to the activation of spinal glial cells. We know that glial cells have CB2 receptors and can be quieted by cannabinoids (Walker 1999; Walter 2003; Nackley 2004). Cannabis holds great promise for treating fibromyalgia because it can lessen central sensitization, in stark contrast to opiates, which stimulate the glial cells and can worsen central sensitization over time (Mao 2000).

The fascia, the connective tissue that surrounds the muscles, is inflamed and painful in fibromyalgia. Fibroblasts, the main cells in the fascia, have both CB1 and CB2 receptors (McPartland 2008). In fibromyalgia these cells overproduce inflammatory chemicals and connective tissue glue, which makes the fascia achy and tight. Cannabinoids treat this by lowering inflammation and lessening the excess production of this connective tissue glue (Garcia-Gonzalez 2009). The gentle stretching of myofascial release increases endocannabinoids—the body's natural anti-inflammatories—which may partly explain why it is so beneficial for fibromyalgia pain (McPartland 2005).

Marijuana as Medicine

Pharmaceutical companies are racing to find ways to produce standardized ingredients and dosing of cannabis. But unfortunately, right now there is nothing "medical" about medical marijuana. There is a black hole between when the doctor signs for a marijuana card (the equivalent of a prescription) and the patient using it medicinally. Most doctors don't know anything about prescribing marijuana, and so can't give guidance on dosing, strains, or usage. Any insight they may have comes not from any medical training but from what they may have learned on their own during youthful experimentation.

Here is a scenario I see frequently: a patient gets a medical marijuana card and goes to a dispensary. There, the employees are the only guide to strain and dose. It's the equivalent of someone walking into a drugstore with a blank prescription and asking the cashier what medicine they should purchase. Some dispensary employees are quite knowledgeable, but often they are just young marijuana enthusiasts who have no idea what to recommend for a fibromyalgia patient. One of my patients who is sixty-five and had never smoked marijuana in her life went to a dispensary and was directed to buy a cookie that contained a very strong strain that was mostly THC. An hour later she started hallucinating and was so scared that she called 911!

FAQ: Is there anyone who should not use medical marijuana?

There are some patients for whom it is absolutely a bad idea. People with active or uncontrolled psychiatric conditions characterized by psychosis should not use marijuana, as it can trigger hallucinations and worsen their symptoms. Marijuana can also increase pulse rate and so should be used with caution in people with heart problems such as atrial fibrillation. Tell your doctor if you have any heart problems prior to trying medical marijuana. Furthermore, anyone with active substance abuse should not use medical marijuana. Marijuana does not have a major potential for addiction, but it can be misused just like any other mind-altering substance.

If you choose to try marijuana, it will be up to you to educate yourself as much as possible if your provider is not able to do so. The most important step is to determine which strain to use, as therapeutic and adverse effects vary widely. There are two cannabis species, and within each family there are hundreds of different strains. *Cannabis sativa* and *Cannabis indica* differ fundamentally in their chemical composition. Indica plants tend to produce more relaxing physical effects and have a sedative quality, while sativa plants are less sedating and more activating. In general, fibromyalgia patients do best with cannabis strains that contain a balanced amount of THC and CBD. One helpful resource is the website www.leafly.com, which is like the Yelp of marijuana, with user reviews on different strains. Interestingly, with marijuana, lower dosages may be better for pain reduction. One study found that while low to moderate doses lowered pain, high doses actually increased it (Wallace 2007).

The next step is to decide the method of use. Smoking anything can cause lung damage, so I recommend avoiding smoking marijuana. Safer methods include vaporizing, ingesting as a food or tincture, or applying topically. Eating is a much slower and inconsistent method due to variations in how the liver processes the marijuana chemicals after they are absorbed though the digestive tract. Inhalation and under-the-tongue absorption of tinctures tend to provide the most consistent responses, because they bypass the digestive system altogether. Many of my patients report great success with topical products, and because very little gets absorbed systemically, this approach does not affect your brain or produce a high.

Methods for Using Marijuana as Medicine

- **Vaporizing:** using a device to heat the marijuana to a very high temperature, producing a cannabinoid-laced vapor to inhale. Vaporizing is healthier than smoking but still produces near-instant effects.

- **Edibles:** food or candy that has been infused with oils from the marijuana plant. Medicating with edibles has a slower onset as it depends on absorption through the digestive system, but the effects are longer-lasting.
- **Tinctures:** a liquid cannabis extract usually made with alcohol or glycerol that is dosed with a dropper under the tongue. This method has slower effects than vaporizing but quicker effects than edibles.
- **Topical:** balms or salves made with marijuana oil rubbed on the skin that act locally as an anti-inflammatory and pain reliever. This method is slower-acting but longer-lasting and produces little to no brain high.

Is Marijuana Safe?

Marijuana is generally considered to be safe, with low toxicity. Unlike opiates, it does not suppress the breathing centers of the brain, so it will not cause you to stop breathing in an overdose. However, we know that just like smoking tobacco, smoking marijuana is harmful to the lungs, so I always recommend a different technique. Cannabis doesn't seem to have significant interactions with any medications, including opioids, although additive effects on motor control and mental status do occur. It reduces reaction time, and studies show that alcohol combined with marijuana leads to significantly higher risks in operating motor vehicles. I always caution my patients who take medical marijuana to only do so when they are going to be in the house all day and never to combine it with alcohol or opiates. It has such positive outcomes for sleep that many of my patients use it just before bed.

To Do Yourself

- Research the laws in your state at www.medicalmarijuana
  .procon.org or Marijuana Policy Project at www.mpp.org.
- For information and user reviews on different strains,
  check out www.leafly.com.
- Read *Cannabis Pharmacy: The Practical Guide to
  Medical Marijuana* by Michael Backes.

To Discuss with Your Health Care Provider

- If medical marijuana is legal in your state, ask your
  HCP if it is something she would support within your
  treatment regimen.

CHAPTER 22

Reduce: Pain from Other Sources

Several painful conditions frequently occur along with fibro-myalgia, including interstitial cystitis, osteoarthritis, and peripheral neuropathy. Treating these can reduce some of the "fire" feeding hypersensitivity and reduce overall pain levels. Irritable bladder syndrome, also called interstitial cystitis, is very common in fibromyalgia. The bladder relies on the rest-and-digest part of the autopilot nervous system, so when that balance is skewed and fight or flight is dominant, bladder function can suffer. Osteoarthritis is common among all people over the age of thirty, but it often hurts more in fibromyalgia due to the brain's increased sensitivity to pain signals. Peripheral neuropathy—pain from damaged nerves—occurs in about one-third of fibromyalgia patients (Oaklander 2013; Giannoc-caro 2014).

Irritable Bladder Syndrome/Interstitial Cystitis

Urinary symptoms, including bladder discomfort, urgency, and frequency of urination, frequently occur in people with fibro-myalgia. Milder bladder symptoms are called irritable bladder syndrome, which is characterized by a frequent urge to urinate and intermittent discomfort. When bladder pain is more severe it is called interstitial cystitis (IC). This condition is character-ized by constant pressure and pain in the bladder area or lower pelvis along with urgency or frequency of urination. There is some evidence that the protective lining of the bladder is bro-ken down, likely due to the effects of a chronic stress response. The breakdown of this mucous lining allows exposure of pain-sensing nerves to the urine and leads to inflammation of the fascia in and around the bladder (Parsons 2007). Pelvic myofas-cial release therapy can help with the symptoms of interstitial cystitis (Weiss 2001; FitzGerald 2012). Treatment also includes limiting irritating substances in the urine: caffeine, alcohol, ar-tificial sweeteners, and spicy foods.

To build up the bladder lining, I recommend fish oil. I also like a supplement called Bladder Ease that contains several ingredients to support the bladder lining, including corn silk, L-arginine, quercetin, and Oregon grape extract. Medications to calm the nerves in the bladder can help reduce pain, like tricyclic antidepressants such as amitriptyline (van Ophoven 2004). Supplementing with L-methylfolate, an activated form of folic acid, has similar benefits. Finally, prescription patches that contain the numbing medicine lidocaine can be placed over the bladder area during pain flares. For severe symptoms it may be helpful to see a urologist or urogynecologist (a urologist who specializes in female bladder issues).

Osteoarthritis

Fibromyalgia causes muscle and fascial pain but does not di-rectly affect the joints. Muscles and joints are connected by fas-cial tissue, and if this is tight it can cause significant pain around the joints. Pain from inside the joints, meanwhile, is usually due to the "wear and tear" arthritis known as osteoarthritis (OA), whether or not you have fibromyalgia. It most commonly man-ifests at the base of the thumbs and the knees, but any joint can be affected. Due to genetics and lifestyle some people start getting symptoms in their thirties, others not until their seventies. They say that if you live long enough you will get osteoarthritis! If you are having a lot of joint pain, talk with your HCP; it may be worthwhile to get an X-ray to assess for osteoarthritis and discuss treatment options. It is also important to rule out rheumatoid arthritis, a different arthritis that is caused by the immune system attacking the joint, causing inflammation.

For osteoarthritis pain I prescribe topical NSAIDs (nonsteroidal anti-inflammatories) (Baraf 2010; Barthel 2009; Roth 2004). Although oral NSAIDs like ibuprofen or naproxen can help, they can make gut leakiness worse, leading to more inflammation in the bloodstream and more pain. I recommend the natural anti-inflammatories in fish oil and turmeric instead. Curcumin, the main ingredient in the yellow spice turmeric, is a potent anti-inflammatory that mitigates OA pain, and omega-3 fatty acids supplements (usually in the form of fish oil) have an anti-inflammatory effect (Belcaro 2010). See chapter 14 for more info about these options. Acupuncture can help ease discomfort as well (Manheimer 2010).

One alternative (but not new) approach to treating arthritis pain is bee venom injections around affected joints (Lee 2008; Lee 2005). Hippocrates wrote about using bee stings for arthritis treatment, and it is a mainstream option outside the United States. Bee venom, a natural product of the honeybee, can be extracted, dried, and added to a sterile solution. A health care provider injects the solution at several places around the joint, causing the same reaction the body has to an actual bee sting, namely an intense activation of the immune system. This releases many chemicals, including those that make a bee sting itchy, hot, and swollen. It also produces anti-inflammatory hormones and mobilizes the immune system to send help to the arthritic joint. As the body heals from the bee sting, it heals the joint as well. I have seen this therapy, both clinically and personally, work wonders for arthritis. Not surprisingly, it can't be used on anyone with an allergy to bee stings, and it must only be performed in a health care provider's office that is prepared to deal with any potentially life-threatening allergic reaction.

Peripheral Neuropathy

Pain from compressed or irritated nerves due to fascial tightness is quite common in fibromyalgia—about half of patients report at least some numbness and burning or prickling sensations (Amris 2010). Typical numbness and tingling is intermittent, occurs in various locations, and tends to be made worse by certain muscle positions or overuse. But when it is constant and always located in the same area, it is called neuropathy, and is often due to nerve damage. Damage to the small pain-sensing nerves is called small fiber neuropathy. Symptoms include persistent tingling or burning sensations, often described as "pins and needles." Patients also describe numbness and loss of sensation, especially in hands and feet, as if they're wearing socks or gloves all the time.

Peripheral Neuropathy Symptoms Survey

If you experience one or more of these symptoms, talk to your HCP about whether you need testing or treatment for peripheral neuropathy.
- Your feet are numb all the time.
- You don't feel pain in your feet, even when you have blisters or injuries.
- You can't feel your feet when you are walking.
- You have trouble feeling heat or cold in your feet or hands.

- Sometimes it feels as if you have socks or gloves on when you don't.
- You feel pins and needles in your feet.
- You have burning, stabbing and/or shooting pains in your feet.
- Your feet or hands get very cold or very hot.

About a third of patients with fibromyalgia have some evidence of nerve damage in their hands and feet, which can be diagnosed by a skin biopsy. A Harvard study reported that 41 percent of biopsy samples taken from fibromyalgia patients showed reduced amounts of small fibers, indicating nerve damage (Oaklander 2013). Another found that a third of patients showed evidence of damage in both the pain-sensing and fight-or-flight nerves. The authors recommended that a "skin biopsy should be considered in the diagnostic work-up of fibromyalgia" (Giannoccaro 2014). This science is still new and it will likely take many years before it is accepted as a routine part of a fibromyalgia medical evaluation.

We don't know exactly why this type of nerve damage occurs in fibromyalgia. It is possible that the chronic activation of fight-or-flight nerves may cause damage to pain-sensing nerves, a phenomenon that has been documented in lab rats (Pertovaara 2013). The biggest question that remains is, why do we find nerve damage in some, but not all, patients with fibromyalgia? Some people may be more vulnerable due to genetics or other conditions that can cause similar damage such as diabetes or nutritional deficiencies.

The best way to protect your nerves is with supplements known to safeguard against damage. It is also critical to make sure to find and treat any other conditions like diabetes or hypothyroidism that can cause nerve damage. Protective supplements include many of the same nutrients used to support energy production in the mitochondria: alpha-lipoic acid, carnitine, and CoQ10 (see chapter 13). Alpha-lipoic acid in particular has been well studied and proven to minimize nerve damage and painful symptoms in diabetes (Ametov 2003; Ziegler 2004, 2006).

Other nerve-protecting supplements include omega-3 fatty acids like those found in fish oil. Fatty acids support the myelin sheath, the protective coating around the nerves. Activated folic acid, B_6, and B_{12} can also ease symptoms and may even promote repair of damaged nerve fibers (Walker 2010). A prescription nutritional supplement called Metanx contains the right proportion of these activated B vitamins. After six months of treatment with Metanx, 80 percent of subjects with diabetic neuropathy reported reduced pain and numbness (Jacobs 2011). This study found that Metanx actually *increased* the number of nerve fibers, possibly reversing the damage done by diabetes. It is generally well tolerated, but occasionally it can cause an upset stomach, so I recommend taking it with meals.

FAQ: Should everyone with fibromyalgia get a skin biopsy to test for small fiber neuropathy?

I recommend a skin biopsy only if you have any symptoms of neuropathy such as burning pain, numbness, or loss of sensation in feet or hands (see the symptom survey on pages 235–236). Talk to your HCP if you are concerned, as you will need to be referred to a neurologist to get diagnosed. The neurologist will often do electrical testing of larger nerve function and may perform a biopsy to count small nerve fibers. If any abnormalities are found, she can do further evaluation to look for potential causes of neuropathy.

To Do Yourself

- For irritable bladder syndrome/interstitial cystitis, try supplements such as Bladder Ease by Vitanica, fish oil, and L-methylfolate.
- For osteoarthritis, consider fish oil and curcumin (turmeric) supplements (refer to chapter 14 for more details).
- If you're interested in bee venom therapy, read more on www.apitherapy.org or talk with a naturopath or acupuncturist.
- Take nerve-protecting supplements (refer to chapter 13 for more details).

To Discuss with Your Health Care Provider

- If you have severe irritable bladder syndrome/interstitial cystitis, request referral to a urologist or urogynecologist.
- If you suspect you have nerve damage, request a referral to a neurologist for evaluation.
- Ask about topical NSAIDs for osteoarthritis pain.

CHAPTER 23

Reduce: Chronic Fatigue Syndrome

M any of my patients tell me they must have chronic fatigue syndrome, because they feel exhausted all the time. This is a common misperception. It is confusing because the terms "fibromyalgia" and "chronic fatigue syndrome" are often—incorrectly—used interchangeably. While there is some overlap, such as fatigue and muscle aches, the two diseases are distinct. Chronic fatigue syndrome is provoked by the immune system; it is not due to an abnormal stress response or sleep condition. Only about 15 percent of my patients with fibromyalgia also truly meet the diagnosis of CFS.

At this point you've worked through the four R's to address every fibromyalgia symptom. But if you have chronic fatigue syndrome in addition to fibromyalgia, you may still have residual fatigue. Improving sleep, reducing the stress response, repairing digestion, rebalancing hormones, and calming inflammation will help, but you will also likely need more specific treatment.

Differences Between Chronic Fatigue Syndrome and Fibromyalgia

Most CFS patients describe a sudden onset of their symptoms, often after a flulike illness. Lingering fatigue, low-grade fevers, sore throat, and swollen lymph nodes point to the immune system as the source. According to one medical review paper, "A severe flu-like illness occurs in most cases of chronic fatigue syndrome (CFS), suggesting that an infection triggers and possibly perpetuates this syndrome" (Chia 2005). About 70 percent of participants in one study reported suffering some type of viral infection before developing CFS (Fluge 2011). Fibromyalgia, on the other hand, usually has a gradual onset, and is not associated with fevers, sore throats, or lymph node swelling.

One of the hallmarks of CFS is dramatically worsened fatigue after any type of exertion, mental or physical. In fact, the Institute of Medicine recently proposed a new name for the condition: systemic exertion intolerance disease (IOM 2015). Their report also supported the idea that CFS is primarily an immune dysfunction due to a preceding viral infection.

In order to be diagnosed with CFS you must have:

1. Clinically unexplained exhaustion lasting six months that is not alleviated by rest and that results in a substantial reduction in level of activity.
2. *And* four or more of the following symptoms:
   - Sore throat
   - Tender lymph nodes in the neck or armpit
   - Muscle pain
   - Joint pain without swelling or redness
   - Headache of a new pattern or severity
   - Non-refreshing sleep
   - Post-exertion malaise (fatigue) lasting longer than twenty-four hours
   - Self-reported impairment in short-term memory or concentration

Certainly anyone with fibromyalgia will recognize some of their symptoms on this list, especially muscle pain, fatigue, and non-refreshing sleep. But while it is rare for a fibromyalgia patient to describe a sore throat or tender lymph nodes, most people with CFS do; 85 percent have a sore throat, 80 percent have swollen and tender lymph nodes, and 75 percent experience ongoing fevers (Straus 1988). Researchers have suggested that "symptoms of painful glands or fever might serve as clinical indicators distinguishing between fibromyalgia and the chronic fatigue syndrome" (Wysenbeek 1991).

Many other findings support the distinction between CFS and fibromyalgia despite some common features. Substance P (a chemical important in the transmission of pain signals in the spinal cord) is elevated in the spinal fluid in fibromyalgia, but normal in CFS (Evengard 1998). CFS often responds to antiviral medications, but fibromyalgia does not (Kendall 2004). While many studies have shown low growth hormone levels in fibromyalgia (as described in chapter 4), CFS has either normal or high levels (Bennett 1997). Also, fibromyalgia patients report a notable improvement in pain and tender points when given growth hormone injections, but CFS patients do not (Moorkens 1998). Sodium oxybate (Xyrem), a medication that increases deep sleep, significantly improves symptoms in fibromyalgia, but not in CFS (Scharf 2003).

Differences Between Chronic Fatigue Syndrome and Fibromyalgia

Chronic Fatigue Syndrome
- Sudden onset of flulike symptoms and viral illness
- Not related to trauma

- Along with fatigue, complaints of sore throat, swollen lymph nodes, and low-grade fever
- Responsiveness to antiviral medications
- Normal growth hormone levels
- Normal substance P levels in spinal cord
- No symptom improvement with medication to induce deep sleep (sodium oxybate)

Fibromyalgia
- Gradual onset of symptoms
- Usually related to trauma
- Along with fatigue, complaints of muscle pain and stiffness
- Nonresponsiveness to antiviral medications
- Low growth hormone levels
- Elevated substance P in spinal cord, indicating abnormal pain processing
- Improvement of symptoms with medication to induce deep sleep (sodium oxybate)

Does a Virus Cause Chronic Fatigue Syndrome?

For the past thirty years, researchers have theorized that CFS is caused by a virus. An alternate name for the condition is myalgic encephalomyelitis, reflecting that hypothesis. The leading virus that has been implicated is called Epstein-Barr virus (EBV), the same one that causes infectious mononucleosis. However, studies have shown conflicting results. The 2015 Institute of Medicine report found "insufficient evidence to conclude that all cases of CFS are caused by EBV infection."

In 2009, a different virus was isolated in the blood of CFS sufferers, and it seemed we had finally found the source. The study got a lot of press, including a feature in *The New York*

Times. It reported that almost all chronic fatigue subjects tested positive for xenotropic murine leukemia virus–related virus (XMRV), compared to only 3.7 percent of healthy people (Lombardi 2009). XMRV is a retrovirus, a member of the same family of viruses as AIDS. But all following research found no evidence of XMRV in CFS blood, and the results of the first study were ultimately determined to be due to lab contamination (Knox 2011; Satterfield 2011). The best theory now is that several different viral infections may trigger the immune dysfunction.

All signs point to CFS as an immune system disease. In fact, an earlier name was CFIDS: chronic fatigue and immune dysfunction syndrome. The immune abnormalities include high levels of the pro-inflammatory cytokines that fight off viruses, chemicals that are well known to cause profound fatigue (Hornig 2015). One cytokine that is elevated in CFS is also high in cases of persistent fatigue after West Nile virus infections (Garcia 2014). Other research found abnormal cytokine patterns, indicating poor communication among certain parts of the immune system, and dysfunctional white blood cells (Broderick 2010).

In particular, the white blood cells called B-lymphocytes have an impaired response to EBV, creating an immune system "blind spot" to this and similar viruses (Loebel 2014; Bradley 2013), allowing the virus to replicate freely. Most of us are exposed to EBV in childhood—a healthy immune system can fight it off but never gets rid of it completely. The virus hibernates in our B-lymphocytes, and when the immune system is not functioning well it can reactivate. This might explain why so many people with CFS test positive for high levels of EBV antibodies; the EBV is not a new cause of the problem but is rather taking advantage of an opportunity given to it by an immune system in distress.

Looked at all together, it seems that CFS likely starts with a viral infection that triggers the immune system to malfunction. The malfunctioning immune system has a blind spot for certain viruses that can now replicate and cause additional problems. So we have to address both the immune system and the uncontrolled viruses to manage the symptoms of CFS.

Treating Chronic Fatigue Syndrome

The most successful treatments are those that alter immune system function in some way. A drug called interferon that stimulates the immune system has shown mild benefit for CFS symptoms (See 1996; Brook 1993). Another, rintatolimod, modulates immune function and produced objective improvement in exercise tolerance and other CFS symptoms. Unfortunately, these effects were not strong enough for the FDA to grant approval for its use for CFS (Strayer 1994, 2012).

An immune system medication that has shown a lot of potential was actually discovered completely by accident. A patient undergoing chemotherapy with rituximab (Rituxan), a drug that kills off B-lymphocytes, had a near-miraculous recovery from her CFS. Further research showed that almost two-thirds of participants who received rituximab improved after only two doses (Fluge 2011). The benefits lasted just for a few months, but it is an exciting new avenue for CFS treatment. This study also confirmed that the related immune dysfunction seems to lie within B-lymphocytes.

Several antiviral medications also seem to be somewhat effective (Lerner 2001, 2007; Watt 2012; Kogelnik 2006). One study found that 50 to 70 percent of CFS patients had reduced symptoms after six months of taking the antiviral valganciclovir (Valcyte) (Montoya 2013).

I have found a two-pronged approach to be the most effective: using antivirals to get the EBV and any other viruses back into hibernation, and simultaneously improving immune function. I base my recommended antiviral regimen on the six-month valganciclovir protocol used in the studies at Stanford University. Antivirals are heavy-duty and require frequent bloodwork to monitor for side effects and toxicity. I also add lauric acid, a natural antiviral derived from coconut oil, marketed as lauricidin (Monolaurin). This supplement has antiviral effects by interfering with the outer membranes of viruses, although it has not been studied specifically for CFS (Hornung 1994; Arora 2011).

In addition to the prescription and natural antivirals, I have patients take two immune-boosting supplements. First, they start on high doses of zinc at 50 mg daily for three months, then 15–25 mg daily. (I recommend taking high-dose zinc for no longer than about three months, as for extended periods it can potentially cause negative health effects, including low iron levels.) They also take thymic protein A (ProBoost), an extract of the thymus gland, one of the key regulators of the immune system. A study of ProBoost found that sixteen of twenty-three patients with CFS experienced improvement of their immune function and symptoms (Rosenbaum 2001).

The diagnosis and treatment of CFS is a rapidly changing field, so I highly recommend working with a health care provider. Keep in mind that if you have both CFS and FM the four R's program will still help you feel better, but you may need to do some extra work to boost your immune system and minimize your viral load.

To Discuss with Your Health Care Provider

- Confirm that you meet the diagnostic criteria for CFS.
- Treat with prescription antivirals. Your HCP can access information about the protocols used at Stanford University at http://med.stanford.edu/chronicfatiguesyndrome/about.html.

ACKNOWLEDGMENTS

I could not have written this book without the support and encouragement of my family. My daughter, Samantha, allowed me time to write and my mother-in-law provided very helpful feedback at many stages of this project. My mom, an author herself, has been an inspiration and provided vital emotional and editorial support. Marrying my husband, Jamie, continues to be the best choice I ever made, and I am forever grateful for his love, advice, and support.

I want to extend my deepest thanks to:

My patients—for your trust in me.

The wonderful healers and teachers who helped me along the way, particularly Gisela Pikarsky, Yuliya Cohen, Ben Benjamin, and John F. Barnes.

The dedicated practitioners and researchers at Oregon Health & Science University, who have taught me so much about treating fibromyalgia, especially Kim Dupree Jones, Robert Bennett, and Cheryl Hryciw.

My agent, Don Fehr, and my excellent editor, Nina Shield, who helped transform my writing from informational to interesting.

Bonnie Hofkin and Emily Brackett for bringing my words to life with their illustrations and graphics.

Frida Kahlo—for inspiration. While struggling with chronic pain, she adorned herself with flowers, took the art world by storm, and attended her final gallery showing while being carried in her bed.

APPENDIX

A Health Care Provider Guide to Fibromyalgia Management

From *The FibroManual: A Complete Fibromyalgia Treatment Guide for You—and Your Doctor* by Ginevra Liptan, MD

As with any chronic illness, successful fibromyalgia treatment requires active patient self-management in addition to targeted medical interventions. The bulk of *The FibroManual* is dedicated to educating patients on lifestyle changes they can make to help themselves. But some key areas of treatment hinge on interventions to improve quality of sleep, reduce peripheral pain generators, and decrease central sensitivity to pain. Some patients may need additional support to address mood, fatigue, and dyscognition (fibrofog). Guidance on these key areas is provided briefly below with citations, along with some clinical pearls. It is my hope that this short guide can be a quick evidence-based reference for you and a starting point to build a successful regimen for your patients with fibromyalgia.

Targeting the primary known physiologic abnormalities should be used to guide effective treatment:

1. **Sympathetic nervous system (SNS) dominance** is seen in heart rate variability studies that show "relentless sympathetic hyperactivity" leading to tense muscles and disturbed sleep (Martínez-Lavín 1998; Kooh 2003).

Treatment:
- Medical intervention: refer for biofeedback therapy, order cranial electrotherapy stimulation.
- Self-management: gentle exercise, yoga, meditation, and other tools to activate the parasympathetic nervous system.

2. **Disrupted sleep patterns**, with inadequate deep sleep and frequent alpha waves, reflect brain mini-arousals (Kooh 2003; Branco 1994). This sleep disturbance significantly contributes to fibromyalgia symptoms of pain and fatigue (Lentz 1999; Moldofsky 1975).

Treatment:
- Medical intervention: find and treat any comorbid sleep disorders, use medications to increase deep sleep.
- Self-management: sleep hygiene.

3. **Peripheral pain generators** include myofascial pain and myofascial trigger points that contribute to both local and overall fibromyalgia pain. Fibromyalgia subjects on average have at least twelve active painful trigger points (Affaitati 2011; Alonso-Blanco 2011).

Treatment:
- Medical intervention: trigger point injections, myofascial therapy, topical NSAIDs, and compounded topical analgesics.
- Self-management: self-treatment of trigger points, stretching, gentle exercise, and yoga.

4. **Central sensitization leading to impaired pain processing** has been well documented in fibromyalgia (Petersel 2011). Central sensitization reflects heightened spinal cord sensitivity to pain signals and impaired descending inhibitory pathways. At the level of the spinal cord, there is enhanced release of glutamate and substance P triggered by activation of dorsal horn glial cells (Watkins 2007; Lee Apr 2011).

Treatment:
- Medical intervention: SNRIs and dopamine agonists to improve descending inhibition of pain. Anticonvulsants, NMDA antagonists, beta-blockers to reduce spinal cord hypersensitivity.
- Self-management: avoiding pain catastrophizing, cognitive-behavioral therapy.

The health care provider guide that follows provides specific information on each of these topics. For ease of understanding, the patient section organizes the approach into four steps: **Rest, Repair, Rebalance,** and **Reduce. Rest** reviews the relaxation response and how to improve sleep quality. **Repair** covers diet, exercise, and myofascial pain. **Rebalance** focuses on lowering inflammation and improving mood. **Reduce** covers central sensitization, fatigue, and dyscognition (fibrofog).

I provide patients with some rules for easing the burden placed on their provider, including asking questions during office visits only, setting up a series of visits to address these various aspects, and respecting the time limits of appointments.

1. Reduce SNS Activation

Techniques patients can use to induce a relaxation response are reviewed extensively. Biofeedback training can be useful; consider referral to PT/OT who does biofeedback. An additional tool is cranial electrotherapy stimulation (CES), microcurrent levels of electricity transmitted between electrodes on each ear that induce a state of relaxation and have been shown to reduce pain and anxiety in fibromyalgia (Lichtbroun 2001). With a prescription, health insurance may cover the cost.

Resources: Cranial electrotherapy stimulation www.alpha -stim.com

2. Improve Sleep Quality

First, evaluate for and treat any comorbid sleep disorders such as restless legs syndrome or obstructive sleep apnea, both of which commonly accompany fibromyalgia (Viola-Saltzman 2010; Gold 2004; May 1993; Shah 2006). Next, eliminate and/or reduce medications that disturb sleep architecture and impair deep sleep, such as opiates and benzodiazepines (Shaw 2005; Dimsdale 2007; Hindmarch 2005). If unable to eliminate offending medications, try to move them away from bedtime hours. The final step is to use medications to reduce nocturnal sympathetic nervous system arousal and promote deep sleep. The most effective are anticonvulsants or $GABA_B$ agonists. Sodium oxybate induces deep sleep via $GABA_B$ activation, and multiple studies have found that it reduces pain and fatigue in fibromyalgia (Staud 2011). Although it showed efficacy, sodium oxybate was unable to gain an indication for fibromyalgia due to concerns of abuse. However, baclofen and tiagabine are also $GABA_B$ agonists with similar but milder benefits (Huang 2009; Brown 2011; Mathias 2001; Walsh 2006). Anticonvulsants such as gabapentin and pregabalin also improve sleep quality (Foldvary-Schaefer 2002; Hindmarch 2005; Roth 2012).

If insomnia is present, a sedative may be needed. The sedating antidepressants trazodone and mirtazapine have positive effects on sleep, with mirtazapine showing specific benefit for fibromyalgia (Mendelson 2005; Schittecatte 2002; Yeephu 2013). Eszopiclone improved fatigue from fibromyalgia and did not negatively affect deep sleep, and zolpidem increased daytime energy (Moldofsky 1996; Drewes 1991; Grönblad 1993). In place of or in addition to sedatives, SNS inhibitors such as antiadrenergics, some muscle relaxants, and antipsychotics can be used. Improved sleep quality and reduced fatigue were seen in FM patients taking the antipsychotic quetiapine, and in others with the muscle relaxant cyclobenzaprine (Hidalgo 2007; Moldofsky 2011).

Clinical pearl: If the patient is on beta-blockers, recommend melatonin since beta-blockers inhibit melatonin release (Stoschitzky 1999).

Medications/Supplements to Improve Sleep

Deep Sleep Promoters	Sedatives	SNS blockers
Anticonvulsants	**"Z-drugs"**	**Muscle relaxants**
• gabapentin 100–1,200 mg (Foldvary-Schaefer 2002) • pregabalin 25–200 mg (Hindmarch 2005; Roth 2012) • topiramate 25–50 mg	• zolpidem 5–10 mg (Moldofsky 1996) • eszopiclone 1–3 mg (Drewes 1991; Grönblad 1996) • zaleplon 5–10 mg	• cyclobenzaprine 5–20 mg (Moldofsky 2011) • tizanidine 2–8 mg
GABA_B agonists	**Sedating antidepressants**	**Antiadrenergics**
• baclofen 5–20 mg (Huang 2009; Brown 2011) • tiagabine 2–8 mg (Mathias 2001; Walsh 2006)	• trazodone 25–200 mg (Mendelson 2005) • amitriptyline 10–30 mg • nortriptyline 10–75 mg • doxepin 1–6 mg • mirtazapine 7.5–45 mg (Schittecatte 2002; Yeephu 2013)	• clonidine 0.1–0.3 mg (Hunt 1986) • guanfacine 1–3 mg • doxazosin 1–8 mg (Boehnlein 2007) • prazosin 1–6 mg
Supplements		**Antipsychotics**
• GABA 250–750 mg plus glycine 1,000 mg • magnesium 300–900 mg (Held 2002)	**THC derivatives**	• ziprasidone 5–20 mg • quetiapine 12.5–100 mg (Hidalgo 2007)
	• dronabinol 2.5–10 mg • nabilone 0.5–1 mg (Ware 2010) • medical marijuana (Feinberg 1975)	o A good starting regimen for someone who is naïve to medications is gabapentin 100–300 mg qhs. o All medications in the table assume qhs dosing. o Patients will usually require at least one agent from the deep sleep promoters to see benefit, and some may need a sedative and/or an SNS blocker as well.
	Supplements	
	• melatonin	

3. Reduce Peripheral Pain Generators

TRIGGER POINT INJECTIONS

Trigger point injections significantly reduce both local and overall fibromyalgia pain (Affaitati 2011; Alonso-Blanco 2011).

MYOFASCIAL RELEASE

Myofascial release, a manual therapy that uses prolonged assisted stretching maneuvers, has been shown to effectively reduce fibromyalgia pain, with benefit at both one and six months post-intervention (Castro-Sánchez 2011, Sep 2011). Myofascial release is performed by specially trained massage and physical therapists.

Resources: www.myofascialrelease.com

TOPICAL NSAIDS

Topical NSAID analgesics can reduce any "hot spots" of localized fibromyalgia pain and are well absorbed into muscular and connective tissues (Argoff 2002; Hsieh 2011). They can attain levels four to seven times greater in muscular tissue versus oral administration, with considerably lower risks of GI side effects (Tegeder 1999). After administration of topical NSAIDs, peak plasma concentrations are 0.2 to 8 percent of concentrations achieved with appropriate oral dosing (Heyneman 2000). Available prescription topical NSAIDs include diclofenac gel, liquid, and patch.

TOPICAL COMPOUNDED ANALGESICS

Topical compounded analgesics usually include an NSAID, ketamine, gabapentin, and clonidine, along with a local anesthetic. The NMDA antagonist ketamine reduces glutamate-evoked afferent discharges and when used topically has minimal systemic absorption (Lynch 2005; Uzaraga 2012; Cairns 2003). One hour after a 10 percent ketamine cream was applied, plasma ketamine levels were undetectable (Finch 2009). Topical clonidine blocks peripheral sympathetic nerve signals that stimulate nociceptors (Campbell 2012).

Rx: Compounded Topical Pain Cream

lidocaine 5 percent (or tetracaine 2 percent)
gabapentin 6 percent
clonidine 0.2 percent
ketamine 10 percent
diclofenac 3 percent (or ketoprofen 10 percent)

Apply 1–2 gm to affected area four times daily as needed.
- Can also be written without ketamine if preferred.
- Prescription will need to be sent to a compounding pharmacy.

Resources: To find a reputable compounding pharmacy, visit www.pccarx.com/contact-us/find-a-compounder.

4. Reduce Central Pain Sensitivity

SNRIs

Duloxetine and milnacipran are effective and FDA-approved for fibromyalgia (Clauw 2008). Off-label usage of venlafaxine is common. Major side effects are sweating, palpitations, and urinary retention.

Clinical pearl: If SNRIs are effective but cause side effect of excess sweating, add low-dose prazosin or clonidine.

DOPAMINE AGONISTS

A randomized controlled double-blind study found that treatment with pramipexole resulted in some improvement in pain, fatigue, and functioning in fibromyalgia (Holman 2005). Side effects included weight loss, nausea, and anxiety and development of an impulse control disorder. Good choice if comorbid RLS.

LOW-DOSE NALTREXONE (LDN)

Naltrexone is an opiate antagonist that in low doses inhibits glial activity in the nervous system and reduces central sensitization. Two Stanford studies demonstrated that LDN reduced fibromyalgia pain, with 57 percent of the participants reporting a significant (one-third) reduction of pain (Younger 2013, 2014). Contraindicated in patients on opiate-based pain medications and is only available as a compounded medication.

LDN Compounded Rx

Low-dose naltrexone 1.5 mg qhs × fourteen days, 3 mg qhs × fourteen days.

If tolerated increase to long-term dose of 4.5 mg qhs.
- Prescription will need to be sent to a compounding pharmacy.

Resources: To find a reputable compounding pharmacy, visit www.pccarx.com/contact-us/find-a-compounder.

ANTICONVULSANTS

Both pregabalin and gabapentin are effective for fibromyalgia pain (Üçeyler Oct 2013; Arnold 2007). They are better tolerated with lower daytime and higher evening dosages and slow dosage titration. Other anticonvulsants such as topiramate may be used instead (Kararizou 2013).

AVOID ACE INHIBITORS

Consider changing from an ACE inhibitor to an ARB. ACE inhibitors interfere with the ACE-dependent degradation of substance P and bradykinin, and increase levels of these pro-inflammatory peptides, potentially exacerbating chronic pain and central sensitization; ARBs do not have this effect (de Mos 2009).

NMDA ANTAGONISTS

Memantine and amantadine reduce pain in conditions characterized by central sensitization (Kleinböhl 2006). A randomized double-blind trial compared a six-month course of memantine (20 mg daily) with placebo and found significant decrease in fibromyalgia pain. Secondary outcomes of depression, cognitive state, and quality of life also improved (Olivan-Blázquez 2014). Titrate dosages up slowly to minimize side effects. Rx: start with 7 mg memantine XR daily and increase slowly to usual effective dosage of 28 mg XR daily. Or use memantine IR 5 mg po daily and increase slowly to usual effective dose of 10 mg bid.

Clinical pearl: Memantine is especially helpful for opiate-induced hyperalgesia.

NON-CARDIOSELECTIVE BETA-BLOCKERS

Non-cardioselective beta-blockers (pindolol and propranolol) reduce fibromyalgia pain through their suppression of SNS amplification of pain signals. Can be used either scheduled or prn for pain flares (Wood 2005).

OPIOIDS

Opioids are not recommended by any practice guidelines, yet they are still frequently prescribed in fibromyalgia (Fitzcharles 2011; Berger 2010). Realistically, until there are better options available, opiate-based pain medications may still be a part of the plan of care for some patients. *The FibroManual* educates patients about the ineffectiveness and negative effects of long-term daily opioids for fibromyalgia, especially opiate-induced hyperalgesia (Lee 2011).

The key to avoiding the negative side effects of opioids is to take them just as needed for occasional pain flares, ideally less than 30 percent of the time (i.e., no more than ten days out of the month). With daily use, those least likely to cause opiate-induced hyperalgesia are tramadol, tapentadol, buprenorphine, or low-dose methadone.

- Tramadol/tapentadol are norepinephrine/serotonin reuptake inhibitors, mild NMDA antagonists, and opiate agonists. Tramadol is the only opiate studied that has been shown to be effective for fibromyalgia pain (Bennett 2003; Russell 2000). A Cochrane review found tapentadol effective for chronic musculoskeletal pain (Santos 2015). One limiting factor is the risk of serotonin syndrome, which is lower with tapentadol as it has only weak serotonin reuptake inhibition.

- Buprenorphine is a partial mu-receptor agonist and kappa and delta antagonist, and so has an "antihyperalgesic effect" that may improve pain in conditions dominated by central sensitization (Koppert 2005).
- Rx: buprenorphine (Butrans) patch 5–20 mcg changed weekly.
- Methadone is an opioid agonist and NMDA antagonist, so at low doses carries less risk of opioid-induced hyperalgesia (Salpeter 2013).

Clinical pearl: If the Butrans patch causes skin irritation, pretreat the intended patch area with a topical corticosteroid.

Tips on Treating Fatigue, Fog, and Comorbid Conditions

FATIGUE

Fatigue generally lessens with improvement of sleep quality, but some patients have residual fatigue that may require treatment. Options include:

- Reducing daytime dosages of sedating medications (pregabalin, gabapentin, and muscle relaxants are the biggest offenders).
- Stimulants such as modafinil or armodafinil. Several case reports show benefit for fatigue due to fibromyalgia (Schwartz 2007, 2010; Schaller 2001).
- Stimulants used for ADD. Patients with coexisting fibromyalgia and ADD treated with stimulants reported improvement in both cognition and fatigue (Young 2007).
- In patients with both fibromyalgia and hypothyroidism, fatigue can be particularly troublesome. In fibromyalgia, there is a blunted TSH response and decreased ability to convert T4 to T3 (Riedel 1998; Tsigos 2002). It may be

helpful to monitor free T3 in addition to TSH and free T4. Consider addition of low-dose T3 to usual T4 regimen.

FIBROFOG

Fibrofog can cause significant impairment, and patients perform poorly in tests of cognitive function, with deficits in memory that mimic about twenty years of aging (Park 2001; Glass 2009). Anecdotal benefits in fibrofog are seen with NMDA antagonists such as memantine, stimulating antidepressants such as bupropion and aripiprazole, and stimulants used for ADD.

PERIPHERAL NEUROPATHY

Peripheral neuropathy is present in 30 to 40 percent of fibromyalgia patients and is of unclear etiology (Oaklander 2013; Giannoccaro 2013; Üçeyler Jun 2013). In addition to standard management of neuropathy, consider a prescription of Metanx, which contains L-methylfolate, pyridoxal 5'-phosphate, and methylcobalamin. After six months of treatment, 80 percent of subjects with neuropathy reported reduced pain and numbness (Jacobs 2011).

Rx: Metanx one cap po bid. If insurance does not cover, patients can get discounted cash price with ninety-day prescriptions sent to Brand Direct Health.

DEPRESSION

Depression is common in fibromyalgia and can be difficult to treat. Several epidemiological studies have associated depression with an impaired ability to metabolize folic acid to L-methylfolate, due to a common polymorphism in methyltetrahydrofolate reductase (MTHFR) (Kelly 2004; Lewis 2006).

One adjunctive approach is to add a prescription form of folic acid called L-methylfolate, which shows benefit when added to standard antidepressant medications (Passeri 1993; Godfrey 1990).

Rx: L-methylfolate (Deplin) 15 mg po daily. If insurance does not cover, patients can get discounted cash price with ninety-day prescriptions sent to Brand Direct Health.

Resources: www.branddirecthealth.com

Health Care Provider Guide References

Affaitati G, Costantini R, Fabrizio A, Lapenna D, Tafuri E, Giamberardino MA. Effects of treatment of peripheral pain generators in fibromyalgia patients. Eur J Pain. 2011 Jan; 15(1):61–69. PubMed PMID: 20889359.

Alonso-Blanco C, Fernández-de-las-Peñas C, Morales-Cabezas M, Zarco-Moreno P, Ge HY, Florez-García M. Multiple active myofascial trigger points reproduce the overall spontaneous pain pattern in women with fibromyalgia and are related to widespread mechanical hypersensitivity. Clin J Pain. 2011 Jun;27(5):405–13. PubMed PMID: 21368661.

Argoff CE. A review of the use of topical analgesics for myofascial pain. Curr Pain Headache Rep. 2002 Oct;6(5):375–78. PubMed PMID: 12207850.

Arnold LM, Goldenberg DL, Stanford SB, Lalonde JK, Sandhu HS, Keck PE Jr, Welge JA, Bishop F, Stanford KE, Hess EV, Hudson JI. Gabapentin in the treatment of fibromyalgia: a randomized, double-blind, placebo-controlled, multicenter trial. Arthritis Rheum. 2007 Apr;56(4):1336–44. PubMed PMID: 17393438.

Bennett RM, Kamin M, Karim R, Rosenthal N. Tramadol and acetaminophen combination tablets in the treatment of fibromyalgia pain: a double-blind, randomized, placebo-controlled study. Am J Med. 2003 May;114(7):537–45. PubMed PMID: 12753877.

Berger A, Sadosky A, Dukes EM, Edelsberg J, Zlateva G, Oster G. Patterns of healthcare utilization and cost in patients with newly diagnosed fibromyalgia. Am J Manag Care. 2010 May;16(5 Suppl):S126–37. PubMed PMID: 20586521.

Boehnlein JK, Kinzie JD. Pharmacologic reduction of CNS noradrenergic activity in PTSD: the case for clonidine and prazosin. J Psychiatr Pract. 2007 Mar;13(2):72–8. PubMed PMID: 17414682.

Branco J, Atalaia A, Paiva T. Sleep cycles and alpha-delta sleep in fibromyalgia syndrome. J Rheumatol. 1994 Jun;21(6): 1113–17. PubMed PMID: 7932424.

Brown MA, Guilleminault C. A review of sodium oxybate and baclofen in the treatment of sleep disorders. Curr Pharm Des. 2011;17(15):1430–35. PubMed PMID: 21476957.

Cairns BE, Svensson P, Wang K, Hupfeld S, Graven-Nielsen T, Sessle BJ, Berde CB, Arendt-Nielsen L. Activation of peripheral NMDA receptors contributes to human pain and rat afferent discharges evoked by injection of glutamate into the masseter muscle. J Neurophysiol. 2003 Oct;90(4):2098–105. PubMed PMID: 12815021.

Campbell CM, Kipnes MS, Stouch BC, Brady KL, Kelly M, Schmidt WK, Petersen KL, Rowbotham MC, Campbell JN. Randomized control trial of topical clonidine for treatment of painful diabetic neuropathy. Pain. 2012 Sep;153(9):1815–23. PubMed PMID: 22683276.

Castro-Sánchez AM, Matarán-Peñarrocha GA, Granero-Molina J, Aguilera-Manrique G, Quesada-Rubio JM, Moreno-

Lorenzo C. Benefits of massage–myofascial release therapy on pain, anxiety, quality of sleep, depression, and quality of life in patients with fibromyalgia. Evid Based Complement Alternat Med. 2011. PubMed PMID: 21234327.

Castro-Sánchez AM, Matarán-Peñarrocha GA, Arroyo-Morales M, Saavedra-Hernández M, Fernández-Sola C, Moreno-Lorenzo C. Effects of myofascial release techniques on pain, physical function, and postural stability in patients with fibromyalgia: a randomized controlled trial. Clin Rehabil. 2011 Sep;25(9):800–813. PubMed PMID: 21673013.

Clauw DJ. Pharmacotherapy for patients with fibromyalgia. J Clin Psychiatry. 2008;69 Suppl 2:25–29. PubMed PMID: 18537460.

de Mos M, Huygen FJ, Stricker BH, Dieleman JP, Sturkenboom MC. The association between ACE inhibitors and the complex regional pain syndrome: suggestions for a neuro-inflammatory pathogenesis of CRPS. Pain. 2009 Apr;142(3):218–24. PubMed PMID: 19195784.

Dimsdale JE, Norman D, DeJardin D, Wallace MS. The effect of opioids on sleep architecture. J Clin Sleep Med. 2007 Feb 15;3(1):33–36. PubMed PMID: 17557450.

Drewes AM, Andreasen A, Jennum P, Nielsen KD. Zopiclone in the treatment of sleep abnormalities in fibromyalgia. Scand J Rheumatol. 1991;20(4):288–93. PubMed PMID: 1925417.

Feinberg I, Jones R, Walker JM, Cavness C, March J. Effects of high dosage delta-9-tetrahydrocannabinol on sleep patterns in man. Clin Pharmacol Ther. 1975 Apr;17(4):458–66. PubMed PMID: 164314.

Finch PM, Knudsen L, Drummond PD. Reduction of allodynia in patients with complex regional pain syndrome: a double-blind placebo-controlled trial of topical ketamine. Pain. 2009 Nov;146(1–2):18–25. PubMed PMID: 19703730.

Fitzcharles MA, Ste-Marie PA, Gamsa A, Ware MA, Shir Y. Opioid use, misuse, and abuse in patients labeled as fibromyalgia. Am J Med. 2011 Oct;124(10):955–60. PubMed PMID: 21962316.

Foldvary-Schaefer N, De Leon Sanchez I, Karafa M, Mascha E, Dinner D, Morris HH. Gabapentin increases slow-wave sleep in normal adults. Epilepsia. 2002 Dec;43(12):1493–97. PubMed PMID: 12460250.

Giannoccaro MP, Donadio V, Incensi A, Avoni P, Liguori R. Small nerve fiber involvement in patients referred for fibromyalgia. Muscle Nerve. 2014 May;49(5):757–59. PubMed PMID: 24469976.

Glass JM. Review of cognitive dysfunction in fibromyalgia: a convergence on working memory and attentional control impairments. Rheum Dis Clin North Am. 2009 May;35(2): 299–311. PubMed PMID: 19647144.

Godfrey PS, Toone BK, Carney MW, Flynn TG, Bottiglieri T, Laundy M, Chanarin I, Reynolds EH. Enhancement of recovery from psychiatric illness by methylfolate. Lancet. 1990 Aug 18;336(8712):392–95. PubMed PMID: 1974941.

Gold AR, Dipalo F, Gold MS, Broderick J. Inspiratory airflow dynamics during sleep in women with fibromyalgia. Sleep. 2004 May 1;27(3):459–66. PubMed PMID: 15164899.

Grönblad M, Nykänen J, Konttinen Y, Järvinen E, Helve T. Effect of zopiclone on sleep quality, morning stiffness, widespread tenderness and pain and general discomfort in primary fibromyalgia patients. A double-blind randomized trial. Clin Rheumatol. 1993 Jun;12(2).186–91. PubMed PMID: 8358976.

Held K, Antonijevic IA, Künzel H, Uhr M, Wetter TC, Golly IC, Steiger A, Murck H. Oral Mg(2+) supplementation reverses age-related neuroendocrine and sleep EEG changes in humans. Pharmacopsychiatry. 2002 Jul;35(4):135–43. PubMed PMID: 12163983.

Heyneman CA, Lawless-Liday C, Wall GC. Oral versus topical NSAIDs in rheumatic diseases: a comparison. Drugs. 2000 Sep;60(3):555–74. Review. PubMed PMID: 11030467.

Hidalgo J, Rico-Villademoros F, Calandre EP. An open-label study of quetiapine in the treatment of fibromyalgia. Prog Neuropsychopharmacol Biol Psychiatry. 2007 Jan 30;31(1):71–77. PubMed PMID: 16889882.

Hindmarch I, Dawson J, Stanley N. A double-blind study in healthy volunteers to assess the effects on sleep of pregabalin compared with alprazolam and placebo. Sleep. 2005 Feb 1;28(2):187–93. PubMed PMID: 16171242.

Holman AJ, Myers RR. A randomized, double-blind, placebo-controlled trial of pramipexole, a dopamine agonist, in patients with fibromyalgia receiving concomitant medications. Arthritis Rheum. 2005 Aug;52(8):2495–505. PubMed PMID: 16052595.

Hsieh LF, Hong CZ, Chern SH, Chen CC. Efficacy and side effects of diclofenac patch in treatment of patients with myofascial pain syndrome of the upper trapezius. J Pain Symptom Manage. 2010 Jan;39(1):116–25. PubMed PMID: 19822404.

Huang YS, Guilleminault C. Narcolepsy: action of two gamma-aminobutyric acid type B agonists, baclofen and sodium oxybate. Pediatr Neurol. 2009 Jul;41(1):9–16. PubMed PMID: 19520267.

Hunt GE, O'Sullivan BT, Johnson GF, Smythe GA. Growth hormone and cortisol secretion after oral clonidine in healthy adults. Psychoneuroendocrinology. 1986;11(3):317–25. PubMed PMID: 3786637

Jacobs AM, Cheng D. Management of diabetic small-fiber neuropathy with combination L-methylfolate, methylcobalamin, and pyridoxal 5'-phosphate. Rev Neurol Dis. 2011;8(1–2):39–47. PubMed PMID: 21769070.

Kararizou E, Anagnostou E, Triantafyllou NI. Dramatic improvement of fibromyalgia symptoms after treatment with topiramate for coexisting migraine. J Clin Psychopharmacol. 2013 Oct;33(5):721–23. PubMed PMID: 23948791.

Kelly CB, McDonnell AP, Johnston TG, Mulholland C, Cooper SJ, McMaster D, Evans A, Whitehead AS. The MTHFR C677T polymorphism is associated with depressive episodes in patients from Northern Ireland. J Psychopharmacol. 2004 Dec;18(4):567–71. PubMed PMID: 15582924.

Kleinböhl D, Görtelmeyer R, Bender HJ, Hölzl R. Amantadine sulfate reduces experimental sensitization and pain in chronic back pain patients. Anesth Analg. 2006 Mar;102(3):840–47. PubMed PMID: 16492838.

Kooh M, Martínez-Lavín M, Meza S, Martín-del-Campo A, Hermosillo AG, Pineda C, Nava A, Amigo MC, Drucker-Colín R. Simultaneous heart rate variability and polysomnographic analyses in fibromyalgia. Clin Exp Rheumatol. 2003 Jul–Aug;21(4):529–30. PubMed PMID: 1294271.

Koppert W, Ihmsen H, Körber N, Wehrfritz A, Sittl R, Schmelz M, Schüttler J. Different profiles of buprenorphine-induced analgesia and antihyperalgesia in a human pain model. Pain. 2005 Nov;118(1–2):15–22. PubMed PMID:16154698.

Lee M, Silverman SM, Hansen H, Patel VB, Manchikanti L. A comprehensive review of opioid-induced hyperalgesia. Pain Physician. 2011 Mar–Apr;14(2):145–61. PubMed PMID: 21412369.

Lee YC, Nassikas NJ, Clauw DJ. The role of the central nervous system in the generation and maintenance of chronic pain in rheumatoid arthritis, osteoarthritis and fibromyalgia. Arthritis Res Ther. 2011 Apr 28;13(2):211. PubMed PMID: 21542893.

Lentz MJ, Landis CA, Rothermel J, Shaver JL. Effects of selective slow wave sleep disruption on musculoskeletal pain and fatigue in middle-aged women. J Rheumatol. 1999 Jul; 26(7):1586–92. PubMed PMID: 10405949.

Lewis SJ, Lawlor DA, Davey Smith G, Araya R, Timpson N, Day IN, Ebrahim S. The thermolabile variant of MTHFR is associated with depression in the British Women's Heart and Health Study and a meta-analysis. Mol Psychiatry. 2006 Apr;11(4):352–60. Review. PubMed PMID: 16402130.

Lichtbroun AS, Raicer MM, Smith RB. The treatment of fibromyalgia with cranial electrotherapy stimulation. J Clin Rheumatol. 2001 Apr;7(2):72–78; discussion 78. PubMed PMID: 17039098.

Lynch ME, Clark AJ, Sawynok J, Sullivan MJ. Topical amitriptyline and ketamine in neuropathic pain syndromes: an open-label study. J Pain. 2005 Oct;6(10):644–49. PubMed PMID: 16202956.

Martínez-Lavín M, Hermosillo AG, Rosas M, Soto ME. Circadian studies of autonomic nervous balance in patients with fibromyalgia: a heart rate variability analysis. Arthritis Rheum. 1998 Nov;41(11):1966–71. PubMed PMID: 9811051.

Mathias S, Wetter TC, Steiger A, Lancel M. The GABA uptake inhibitor tiagabine promotes slow wave sleep in normal elderly subjects. Neurobiol Aging. 2001 Mar–Apr;22(2):247–53. PubMed PMID: 11182474.

May KP, West SG, Baker MR, Everett DW. Sleep apnea in male patients with the fibromyalgia syndrome. Am J Med. 1993 May;94(5):505–8. PubMed PMID: 8498395.

Mendelson WB. A review of the evidence for the efficacy and safety of trazodone in insomnia. J Clin Psychiatry. 2005 Apr;66(4):469–76. PubMed PMID: 1581678.

Moldofsky H, Scarisbrick P, England R, Smythe H. Musculos-ketal symptoms and non-REM sleep disturbance in patients with "fibrositis syndrome" and healthy subjects. Psychosom Med. 1975 Jul–Aug;37(4):341–51. PubMed PMID: 169541.

Moldofsky H, Lue FA, Mously C, Roth-Schechter B, Reynolds WJ. The effect of zolpidem in patients with fibromyalgia: a dose ranging, double blind, placebo controlled, modified crossover study. J Rheumatol. 1996 Mar;23(3):529–33. PubMed PMID: 8832997.

Moldofsky H, Harris HW, Archambault WT, Kwong T, Leder-man S. Effects of bedtime very low dose cyclobenzaprine on symptoms and sleep physiology in patients with fibromyalgia syndrome: a double-blind randomized placebo-controlled study. J Rheumatol. 2011 Dec;38(12):2653–63. PubMed PMID: 21885490.

Oaklander AL, Herzog ZD, Downs HM, Klein MM. Objective evidence that small-fiber polyneuropathy underlies some ill-nesses currently labeled as fibromyalgia. Pain. 2013 Nov; 154(11):2310–16. PubMed PMID: 23748113.

Olivan-Blázquez B, Herrera-Mercadal P, Puebla-Guedea M, Pérez-Yus MC, Andrés E, Fayed N, López Del Hoyo Y, Magallon R, Roca M, Garcia-Campayo J. Efficacy of memantine in the treatment of fibromyalgia: a double-blind, randomised, controlled trial with 6-month follow-up. Pain. 2014 Dec; 155(12):2517–25. PubMed PMID: 25218600.

Park DC, Glass JM, Minear M, Crofford LJ. Cognitive function in fibromyalgia patients. Arthritis Rheum. 2001 Sep;44(9): 2125–33. PubMed PMID: 11592377.

Passeri M, Cucinotta D, Abate G, Senin U, Ventura A, Stramba Badiale M, Diana R, La Greca P, Le Grazie C. Oral 5'-methyltetrahydrofolic acid in senile organic mental disorders with depression: results of a double-blind multicenter study. Aging (Milano). 1993 Feb;5(1):63–71. PubMed PMID: 8257478.

Petersel DL, Dror V, Cheung R. Central amplification and fibromyalgia: disorder of pain processing. J Neurosci Res. 2011 Jan;89(1):29–34. Review. PubMed PMID: 20936697.

Riedel W, Layka H, Neeck G. Secretory pattern of GH, TSH, thyroid hormones, ACTH, cortisol, FSH, and LH in patients with fibromyalgia syndrome following systemic injection of the relevant hypothalamic-releasing hormones. Z Rheumatol. 1998;57 Suppl 2:81–87. PubMed PMID: 10025090.

Roth T, Lankford DA, Bhadra P, Whalen E, Resnick EM. Effect of pregabalin on sleep in patients with fibromyalgia and sleep maintenance disturbance: a randomized, placebo-controlled, 2-way crossover polysomnography study. Arthritis Care Res (Hoboken). 2012 Apr;64(4):597–606. PubMed PMID: 22232085.

Russell IJ, Kamin M, Bennett RM, Schnitzer TJ, Green JA, Katz WA. Efficacy of tramadol in treatment of pain in fibromyalgia.

J Clin Rheumatol. 2000 Oct;6(5):250–57. PubMed PMID: 19078481.

Salpeter SR, Buckley JS, Bruera E. The use of very-low-dose methadone for palliative pain control and the prevention of opioid hyperalgesia. J Palliat Med. 2013 Jun;16(6):616–22. PubMed PMID: 23556990.

Santos J, Alarcão J, Fareleira F, Vaz-Carneiro A, Costa J. Tapentadol for chronic musculoskeletal pain in adults. Cochrane Database Syst Rev. 2015 May 27;5:CD009923. PubMed PMID: 26017279.

Schaller JL, Behar D. Modafinil in fibromyalgia treatment. J Neuropsychiatry Clin Neurosci. 2001 Fall;13(4):530–31. PubMed PMID: 11748325.

Schittecatte M, Dumont F, Machowski R, Cornil C, Lavergne F, Wilmotte J. Effects of mirtazapine on sleep polygraphic variables in major depression. Neuropsychobiology. 2002;46(4): 197–201. PubMed PMID: 12566938.

Schwartz TL, Rayancha S, Rashid A, Chlebowksi S, Chilton M, Morell M. Modafinil treatment for fatigue associated with fibromyalgia. J Clin Rheumatol. 2007 Feb;13(1):52. PubMed PMID: 17278955.

Schwartz TL, Siddiqui UA, Raza S, Morell M. Armodafinil for fibromyalgia fatigue. Ann Pharmacother. 2010 Jul–Aug;44(7–8):1347–8. PubMed PMID: 20551299.

Shah MA, Feinberg S, Krishnan E. Sleep-disordered breathing among women with fibromyalgia syndrome. J Clin Rheumatol. 2006 Dec;12(6):277–81. PubMed PMID: 17149057.

Shaw IR, Lavigne G, Mayer P, Choinière M. Acute intravenous administration of morphine perturbs sleep architecture in healthy pain-free young adults: a preliminary study. Sleep. 2005 Jun 1;28(6):677–82 PubMed PMID: 16477954.

Staud R. Sodium oxybate for the treatment of fibromyalgia. Expert Opin Pharmacother. 2011 Aug;12(11):1789–98. PubMed PMID: 21679091.

Stoschitzky K, Sakotnik A, Lercher P, Zweiker R, Maier R, Liebmann P, Lindner W. Influence of beta-blockers on melatonin release. Eur J Clin Pharmacol. 1999 Apr;55(2):111–5. PubMed PMID: 10335905.

Tegeder I, Muth-Selbach U, Lötsch J, Rüsing G, Oelkers R, Brune K, Meller S, Kelm GR, Sörgel F, Geisslinger G. Application of microdialysis for the determination of muscle and subcutaneous tissue concentrations after oral and topical ibuprofen administration. Clin Pharmacol Ther. 1999 Apr;65(4):357–68. PubMed PMID: 10223771.

Tsigos C, Chrousos GP. Hypothalamic-pituitary-adrenal axis, neuroendocrine factors and stress. J Psychosom Res. 2002 Oct;53(4):865–71. Review. PubMed PMID: 12377295.

Üçeyler N, Zeller D, Kahn AK, Kewenig S, Kittel-Schneider S, Schmid A, Casanova-Molla J, Reiners K, Sommer C. Small fibre pathology in patients with fibromyalgia syndrome. Brain. 2013 Jun;136(Pt 6):1857–67. PubMed PMID: 23474848.

Üçeyler N, Sommer C, Walitt B, Häuser W. Anticonvulsants for fibromyalgia. Cochrane Database Syst Rev. 2013 Oct 16;10:CD010782. PubMed PMID: 24129853.

Uzaraga I, Gerbis B, Holwerda E, Gillis D, Wai E. Topical amitriptyline, ketamine, and lidocaine in neuropathic pain caused by radiation skin reaction: a pilot study. Support Care Cancer. 2012 Jul;20(7):1515–24. PubMed PMID: 21847539.

Viola-Saltzman M, Watson NF, Bogart A, Goldberg J, Buchwald D. High prevalence of restless legs syndrome among patients with fibromyalgia: a controlled cross-sectional study. J Clin Sleep Med. 2010 Oct 15;6(5):423–27. PubMed PMID: 20957840.

Walsh JK, Perlis M, Rosenthal M, Krystal A, Jiang J, Roth T. Tiagabine increases slow-wave sleep in a dose-dependent fashion without affecting traditional efficacy measures in adults with primary insomnia. J Clin Sleep Med. 2006 Jan 15;2(1):35–41. PubMed PMID: 17557435.

Ware MA, Fitzcharles MA, Joseph L, Shir Y. The effects of nabilone on sleep in fibromyalgia: results of a randomized controlled trial. Anesth Analg. 2010 Feb 1;110(2):604–10. PubMed PMID: 20007734.

Watkins LR, Hutchinson MR, Ledeboer A, Wieseler-Frank J, Milligan ED, Maier SF. Glia as the "bad guys": implications for improving clinical pain control and the clinical utility of opioids. Brain Behav Immun. 2007 Feb;21(2):131–46. PubMed PMID: 17175134.

Wood PB, Kablinger AS, Caldito GS. Open trial of pindolol in the treatment of fibromyalgia. Ann Pharmacother. 2005 Nov;39(11):1812–6. PubMed PMID: 16219901.

Yeephu S, Suthisisang C, Suttiruksa S, Prateepavanich P, Limampai P, Russell IJ. Efficacy and safety of mirtazapine in fibromyalgia syndrome patients: a randomized placebo-controlled pilot study. Ann Pharmacother. 2013 Jul–Aug; 47(7–8):921–32. PubMed PMID: 23737510.

Young JL, Redmond JC. Fibromyalgia, chronic fatigue, and adult attention deficit hypcractivity disorder in the adult: a case study. Psychopharmacol Bull. 2007;40(1):118–26. PubMed PMID: 17285103.

Younger J, Noor N, McCue R, Mackey S. Low-dose naltrexone for the treatment of fibromyalgia: findings of a small, randomized, double-blind, placebo-controlled, counterbalanced, crossover trial assessing daily pain levels. Arthritis Rheum. 2013 Feb;65(2):529–38. PubMed PMID: 23359310.

Younger J, Parkitny L, McLain D. The use of low-dose naltrexone (LDN) as a novel anti-inflammatory treatment for chronic pain. Clin Rheumatol. 2014 Apr;33(4):451–59. PubMed PMID: 24526250.

REFERENCES

Introduction

Gracely RH, Petzke F, Wolf JM, Clauw DJ. Functional magnetic resonance imaging evidence of augmented pain processing in fibromyalgia. Arthritis Rheum. 2002 May;46(5):1333–43. PubMed PMID: 12115241.

Hadker N, Garg S, Chandran AB, Crean SM, McNett MM, Silverman SL. Efficient practices associated with diagnosis, treatment and management of fibromyalgia among primary care physicians. Pain Res Manag. 2011 Nov–Dec;16(6):440–44. PubMed PMID: 22184554.

Martínez-Lavín M, Amigo MC, Coindreau J, Canoso J. Fibromyalgia in Frida Kahlo's life and art. Arthritis Rheum. 2000 Mar;43(3):708–9. PubMed PMID: 10728769.

Perrot S, Choy E, Petersel D, Ginovker A, Kramer E. Survey of physician experiences and perceptions about the diagnosis and treatment of fibromyalgia. BMC Health Serv Res. 2012 Oct 10;12:356. PubMed PMID: 23051101.

Chapter 1. Figuring Out Fibromyalgia for Myself

Jones KD, Liptan GL. Exercise interventions in fibromyalgia: clinical applications from the evidence. Rheum Dis Clin North Am. 2009 May;35(2):373–91. PubMed PMID: 19647149.

Jones KD, Kindler LL, Liptan GL. Self-management in fibromyalgia. J Clin Rheumatol Musculoskelet Med. 2012 Jul;3(1): 59–68.

Liptan GL. Fascia: a missing link in our understanding of the pathology of fibromyalgia. J Bodyw Mov Ther. 2010 Jan;14(1):3–12. PubMed PMID: 20006283.

Liptan GL, Mist S, Wright C, Arzt A, Jones KD. A pilot study of myofascial release therapy compared to Swedish massage in fibromyalgia. J Bodyw Mov Ther. 2013 Jul;17(3):365–70. PubMed PMID: 23768283.

Chapter 2. What Fibromyalgia Is—and Isn't

Behm FG, Gavin IM, Karpenko O, Lindgren V, Gaitonde S, Gashkoff PA, Gillis BS. Unique immunologic patterns in fibromyalgia. BMC Clin Pathol. 2012 Dec 17;12:25. PubMed PMID: 23245186.

CDC (Centers for Disease Control and Prevention). CDC provides estimate of Americans diagnosed with Lyme disease each year. 2013 Aug 19. http://www.cdc.gov/media/releases /2013/p0819-lyme-disease.html.

Dinerman H, Steere AC. Lyme disease associated with fibromyalgia. Ann Intern Med. 1992 Aug 15;117(4):281–85. PubMed PMID: 1637022.

Haliloglu S, Carlioglu A, Akdeniz D, Karaaslan Y, Kosar A. Fibromyalgia in patients with other rheumatic diseases: prevalence and relationship with disease activity. Rheumatol Int. 2014 Sep;34(9)1275–80. PubMed PMID: 24589726.

Lawrence RC, Helmick CG, Arnett FC, Deyo RA, Felson DT, Giannini EH, Heyse SP, Hirsch R, Hochberg MC, Hunder GG,

Liang MH, Pillemer SR, Steen VD, Wolfe F. Estimates of the prevalence of arthritis and selected musculoskeletal disorders in the United States. Arthritis Rheum. 1998 May;41(5):778–99. PubMed PMID: 9588729.

Mease PJ, Gibofksy A, Clark M. Diagnosis, neurobiology, pathophysiology and treatment of fibromyalgia for primary care physicians. MD Magazine. 2011 Aug 23. www.hcplive .com/publications/pain-management/2011/july-2011 /Diagnosis-Neurobiology-Pathophysiology-and-Treatment -of-Fibromyalgia-for-Primary-Care-Physicians.

Middleton GD, McFarlin JE, Lipsky PE. The prevalence and clinical impact of fibromyalgia in systemic lupus erythe-matosus. Arthritis Rheum. 1994 Aug;37(8):1181–88. PMID: 8053957.

Sturgill J, McGee E, Menzies V. Unique cytokine signature in the plasma of patients with fibromyalgia. J Immunol Res. 2014;2014:938576. PubMed PMID: 24741634.

White KP, Speechley M, Harth M, Ostbye T. The London Fibro-myalgia Epidemiology Study: the prevalence of fibromyalgia syndrome in London, Ontario. J Rheumatol. 1999 Jul;26(7): 1570–76. PubMed PMID: 10405947.

Wolfe F, Smythe HA, Yunus MB, Bennett RM, Bombardier C, Goldenberg DL, Tugwell P, Campbell SM, Abeles M, Clark P, et al. The American College of Rheumatology 1990 criteria for the classification of fibromyalgia. Report of the Multicenter Criteria Committee. Arthritis Rheum. 1990 Feb;33(2):160–72. PubMed PMID: 2306288.

Wolfe F, Clauw DJ, Fitzcharles MA, Goldenberg DL, Häuser W, Katz RS, Mease P, Russell AS, Russell IJ, Winfield JB. Fibromy-algia criteria and severity scales for clinical and epidemiologi-cal studies; a modification of the ACR Preliminary Diagnostic

Criteria for Fibromyalgia. J Rheumatol. 2011 Jun;38(6):1113–22. PubMed PMID: 21285161.

Chapter 3. The Chain Reaction That Causes Fibromyalgia

Al-Allaf AW, Dunbar KL, Hallum NS, Nosratzadeh B, Templeton KD, Pullar T. A case-control study examining the role of physical trauma in the onset of fibromyalgia syndrome. Rheumatology (Oxford). 2002 Apr;41(4):450–53. PubMed PMID: 11961177.

Amital D, Fostick L, Polliack ML, Segev S, Zohar J, Rubinow A, Amital H. Posttraumatic stress disorder, tenderness, and fibromyalgia syndrome: are they different entities? J Psychosom Res. 2006 Nov;61(5):663–69. PubMed PMID 17084145.

Arnold LM, Hudson JI, Hess EV, Ware AE, Fritz DA, Auchenbach MB, Starck LO, Keck PE Jr. Family study of fibromyalgia. Arthritis Rheum. 2004 Mar;50(3):944–52. PubMed PMID: 15022338.

Barbosa FR, Matsuda JB, Mazucato M, de Castro França S, Zingaretti SM, da Silva LM, Martinez-Rossi NM, Júnior MF, Marins M, Fachin AL. Influence of catechol-O-methyltransferase (COMT) gene polymorphisms in pain sensibility of Brazilian fibromyalgia patients. Rheumatol Int. 2012 Feb;32(2):427–30. PubMed PMID: 21120493.

Bou-Holaigah I, Calkins H, Flynn JA, Tunin C, Chang HC, Kan JS, Rowe PC. Provocation of hypotension and pain during upright tilt table testing in adults with fibromyalgia. Clin Exp Rheumatol. 1997 May–Jun;15(3):239–46. PubMed PMID: 9177917.

Buskila D, Neumann L, Vaisberg G, Alkalay D, Wolfe F. Increased rates of fibromyalgia following cervical spine injury. A controlled study of 161 cases of traumatic injury. Arthritis Rheum. 1997 Mar;40(3):446–52. PubMed PMID: 9082932.

Cohen H, Neumann L, Glazer Y, Ebstein RP, Buskila D. The relationship between a common catechol-O-methyltransferase (COMT) polymorphism val(158) met and fibromyalgia. Clin Exp Rheumatol. 2009 Sep–Oct;27(5 Suppl 56):S51–56. PubMed PMID: 20074440.

Desmeules J, Chabert J, Rebsamen M, Rapiti E, Piguet V, Besson M, Dayer P, Cedraschi C. Central pain sensitization, COMT Val158Met polymorphism, and emotional factors in fibromyalgia. J Pain. 2014 Feb;15(2):129–35. PubMed PMID: 24342707.

Dinerman H, Steere AC. Lyme disease associated with fibromyalgia. Ann Intern Med. 1992 Aug 15;117(4):281–85. PubMed PMID: 1637022.

Donello JE, Guan Y, Tian M, Cheevers CV, Alcantara M, Cabrera S, Raja SN, Gil DW. A peripheral adrenoceptor-mediated sympathetic mechanism can transform stress-induced analgesia into hyperalgesia. Anesthesiology. 2011 Jun;114(6):1403–16. PubMed PMID: 21540738.

Elenkov IJ, Wilder RL, Chrousos GP, Vizi ES. The sympathetic nerve—an integrative interface between two supersystems: the brain and the immune system. Pharmacol Rev. 2000 Dec;52(4):595–638. PubMed PMID: 11121511.

Greenfield S, Fitzcharles MA, Esdaile JM. Reactive fibromyalgia syndrome. Arthritis Rheum. 1992 Jun;35(6):678–81. PubMed PMID: 1599521.

Holman AJ. Positional cervical spinal cord compression and fibromyalgia: a novel comorbidity with important diagnostic and treatment implications. J Pain. 2008 Jul;9(7):613–22. PubMed PMID: 18499527.

Hryciw CA, Holman AJ. Positional cervical spinal cord compression as a comorbidity in patients with fibromyalgia (FM): findings from a one-year retrospective study at an FM referral university. Myopain 2010, abstract 36.

Lerma C, Martinez A, Ruiz N, Vargas A, Infante O, Martinez-Lavin M. Nocturnal heart rate variability parameters as potential fibromyalgia biomarker: correlation with symptoms severity. Arthritis Res Ther. 2011;13(6):R185. PubMed PMID: 22087605.

Maekawa K, Twe C, Lotaif A, Chiappelli F, Clark GT. Function of beta-adrenergic receptors on mononuclear cells in female patients with fibromyalgia. J Rheumatol. 2003 Feb;30(2):364–68. PubMed PMID: 12563697.

Martinez-Jauand M, Sitges C, Rodríguez V, Picornell A, Ramon M, Buskila D, Montoya P. Pain sensitivity in fibromyalgia is associated with catechol-O-methyltransferase (COMT) gene. Eur J Pain. 2013 Jan;17(1):16–27. PubMed PMID: 22528689.

Martínez-Lavín M. Fibromyalgia: When distress becomes (un)sympathetic pain. Pain Res Treat. 2012;2012:981565. PubMed PMID: 22110948.

Martínez-Lavín M, Hermosillo AG, Rosas M, Soto ME. Circadian studies of autonomic nervous balance in patients with fibromyalgia: a heart rate variability analysis. Arthritis Rheum. 1998 Nov;41(11):1966–71. PubMed PMID: 9811051.

Vargas-Alarcón G, Fragoso JM, Cruz-Robles D, Vargas A, Martinez A, Lao-Villadóniga JI, García-Fructuoso F, Vallejo M, Martínez-Lavín M. Association of adrenergic receptor gene polymorphisms with different fibromyalgia syndrome domains. Arthritis Rheum. 2009 Jul;60(7):2169–73. PubMed PMID: 19565482.

Walker EA, Keegan D, Gardner G, Sullivan M, Katon WJ, Bernstein D. Psychosocial factors in fibromyalgia compared with rheumatoid arthritis: I. Psychiatric diagnoses and functional disability. Psychosom Med. 1997 Nov–Dec;59(6):565–71. PubMed PMID: 9407573.

White KP, Speechley M, Harth M, Ostbye T. The London Fibromyalgia Epidemiology Study: the prevalence of fibromyalgia syndrome in London, Ontario. J Rheumatol. 1999 Jul;26(7): 1570–76. PubMed PMID: 10405947.

Xiao Y, He W, Russell IJ. Genetic polymorphisms of the beta2-adrenergic receptor relate to guanosine protein-coupled stimulator receptor dysfunction in fibromyalgia syndrome. J Rheumatol. 2011 Jun;38(6):1095–103. PubMed PMID: 21406495.

Chapter 4. Blocking the Fibromyalgia Chain Reaction

Anders C, Sprott H, Scholle HC. Surface EMG of the lumbar part of the erector trunci muscle in patients with fibromyalgia. Clin Exp Rheumatol. 2001 Jul–Aug;19(4):453–55. PubMed PMID: 11491504.

Bachasson D, Guinot M, Wuyam B, Favre-Juvin A, Millet GY, Levy P, Verges S. Neuromuscular fatigue and exercise capacity in fibromyalgia syndrome. Arthritis Care Res (Hoboken). 2013 Mar;65(3):432–40. PubMed PMID: 22965792.

Bagge E, Bengtsson BA, Carlsson L, Carlsson J. Low growth hormone secretion in patients with fibromyalgia—a preliminary report on 10 patients and 10 controls. J Rheumatol. 1998 Jan;25(1):145–48. PubMed PMID: 9458218.

Bazzichi L, Dini M, Rossi A, Corbianco S, De Feo P, Giacomelli C, Zirafa C, Ferrari C, Rossi B, Bombardieri S. Muscle modifications in fibromyalgic patients revealed by surface electromyography (SEMG) analysis. BMC Musculoskelet Disord. 2009 Apr 15;10:36. PubMed PMID: 19368705.

Bennett RM, Clark SC, Walczyk J. A randomized, double-blind, placebo-controlled study of growth hormone in the treatment of fibromyalgia. Am J Med. 1998 Mar;104(3):227–31. PubMed PMID: 9552084.

Branco J, Atalaia A, Paiva T. Sleep cycles and alpha-delta sleep in fibromyalgia syndrome. J Rheumatol. 1994 Jun;21(6):1113–17. PubMed PMID: 7932424.

Cuatrecasas G, Riudavets C, Güell MA, Nadal A. Growth hormone as concomitant treatment in severe fibromyalgia associated with low IGF-1 serum levels. A pilot study. BMC Musculoskelet Disord. 2007 Nov 30;8:119. PubMed PMID: 18053120.

Elenkov IJ, Wilder RL, Chrousos GP, Vizi ES. The sympathetic nerve—an integrative interface between two supersystems: the brain and the immune system. Pharmacol Rev. 2000 Dec;52(4):595–638. PubMed PMID: 11121511.

Felig, Phillip, Baxter JD, Frohman LA. Endocrinology and metabolism. Third edition. New York: McGraw-Hill, 1995.

Gerdle B, Söderberg K, Salvador Puigvert L, Rosendal L, Larsson B. Increased interstitial concentrations of pyruvate and lactate in the trapezius muscle of patients with fibromyalgia: a microdialysis study. J Rehabil Med. 2010 Jul;42(7):679–87. PubMed PMID: 20603699.

Gerdle B, Forsgren MF, Bengtsson A, Leinhard OD, Sören B, Karlsson A, Brandejsky V, Lund E, Lundberg P. Decreased muscle concentrations of ATP and PCR in the quadriceps muscle of fibromyalgia patients—a 31P-MRS study. Eur J Pain. 2013 Sep;17(8):1205–15. PubMed PMID: 23364928.

Ghilardi JR, Freeman KT, Jimenez-Andrade JM, Coughlin KA, Kaczmarska MJ, Castaneda-Corral G, Bloom AP, Kuskowski MA, Mantyh PW. Neuroplasticity of sensory and sympathetic nerve fibers in a mouse model of a painful arthritic joint. Arthritis Rheum. 2012 Jul;64(7):2223–32. PubMed PMID: 22246649.

Haack M, Sanchez E, Mullington JM. Elevated inflammatory markers in response to prolonged sleep restriction are associated with increased pain experience in healthy volunteers. Sleep. 2007 Sep 1;30(9):1145–52. PubMed PMID: 17910386.

Harding SM. Sleep in fibromyalgia patients: subjective and objective findings. Am J Med Sci. 1998 Jun;315(6):367–76. PubMed PMID: 9638893.

Jones KD, Deodhar P, Lorentzen A, Bennett RM, Deodhar AA. Growth hormone perturbations in fibromyalgia: a review. Semin Arthritis Rheum. 2007 Jun;36(6):357–79. PubMed PMID: 17224178.

Klingler W, Velders M, Hoppe K, Pedro M, Schleip R. Clinical relevance of fascial tissue and dysfunctions. Curr Pain Headache Rep. 2014;18(8):439. PubMed PMID: 24962403.

Kokebie R, Aggarwal R, Kahn S, Kartz RS. Muscle tension is increased in fibromyalgia: use of a pressure gauge. Abstract 1935, American College of Rheumatology 2008 Annual Scientific Meeting, San Francisco, California. 2008 Oct 24–29.

Kooh M, Martínez-Lavín M, Meza S, Martín-del-Campo A, Hermosillo AG, Pineda C, Nava A, Amigo MC, Drucker-Colín R. Simultaneous heart rate variability and polysomnographic analyses in fibromyalgia. Clin Exp Rheumatol. 2003 Jul–Aug;21(4):529–30. PubMed PMID: 1294271.

Landis CA, Lentz MJ, Rothermel J, Riffle SC, Chapman D, Buchwald D, Shaver JL. Decreased nocturnal levels of prolactin and growth hormone in women with fibromyalgia. J Clin Endocrinol Metab. 2001 Apr;86(4):1672–78. PubMed PMID: 11297602.

Leal-Cerro A, Povedano J, Astorga R, Gonzalez M, Silva H, Garcia-Pesquera F, Casanueva FF, Dieguez C. The growth hormone (GH)-releasing hormone-GH-insulin-like growth factor-1 axis in patients with fibromyalgia syndrome. J Clin Endocrinol Metab. 1999 Sep;84(9):3378–81. PubMed PMID: 10487713.

Lentz MJ, Landis CA, Rothermel J, Shaver JL. Effects of selective slow wave sleep disruption on musculoskeletal pain and fatigue in middle-aged women. J Rheumatol. 1999 Jul;26(7):1586–92. PubMed PMID: 10405949.

Lerma C, Martinez A, Ruiz N, Vargas A, Infante O, Martinez-Lavin M. Nocturnal heart rate variability parameters as potential fibromyalgia biomarker: correlation with symptoms severity. Arthritis Res Ther. 2011;13(6):R185. PubMed PMID: 22087605.

Longo G, Osikowicz M, Ribeiro-da-Silva A. Sympathetic fiber sprouting in inflamed joints and adjacent skin contributes to pain-related behavior in arthritis. J Neurosci. 2013 Jun 12; 33(24):10066–74. PubMed PMID: 23761902.

Mahdi AA, Fatima G, Das SK, Verma NS. Abnormality of circadian rhythm of serum melatonin and other biochemical parameters in fibromyalgia syndrome. Indian J Biochem Biophys. 2011 Apr;48(2):82–87. PubMed PMID: 21682138.

Moldofsky H. The significance of the sleeping-waking brain for the understanding of widespread musculoskeletal pain and fatigue in fibromyalgia syndrome and allied syndromes. Joint Bone Spine. 2008 Jul;75(4):397–402. PubMed PMID: 18456536.

Park JH, Phothimat P, Oates CT, Hernanz-Schulman M, Olsen NJ. Use of P-31 magnetic resonance spectroscopy to detect metabolic abnormalities in muscles of patients with fibromyalgia. Arthritis Rheum. 1998 Mar;41(3):406–13. PubMed PMID: 9506567.

Petersel DL, Dror V, Cheung R. Central amplification and fibromyalgia: disorder of pain processing. J Neurosci Res. 2011 Jan;89(1):29–34. PubMed PMID: 20936697.

Riedel W, Layka H, Neeck G. Secretory pattern of GH, TSH, thyroid hormones, ACTH, cortisol, FSH, and LH in patients with fibromyalgia syndrome following systemic injection of the relevant hypothalamic-releasing hormones. Z Rheumatol. 1998;57 Suppl 2:81–87. PubMed PMID: 10025090.

Russell IJ, Orr MD, Littman B, Vipraio GA, Alboukrek D, Michalek JE, Lopez Y, MacKillip F. Elevated cerebrospinal fluid levels of substance P in patients with the fibromyalgia syndrome. Arthritis Rheum. 1994 Nov;37(11):1593–601. PubMed PMID: 7526868.

Rüster M, Franke S, Späth M, Pongratz DE, Stein G, Hein GE. Detection of elevated N epsilon-carboxymethyllysine levels in muscular tissue and in serum of patients with fibromyalgia. Scand J Rheumatol. 2005 Nov–Dec;34(6):460–63. PubMed PMID: 16393769.

Sato J, Perl ER. Adrenergic excitation of cutaneous pain receptors induced by peripheral nerve injury. Science. 1991 Mar 29;251(5001):1608–10. PubMed PMID: 2011742.

Schleip R, Klingler W, Lehmann-Horn F. Active fascial contractility: fascia may be able to contract in a smooth muscle-like manner and thereby influence musculoskeletal dynamics. Med Hypotheses. 2005;65(2):273–77. PubMed PMID: 15922099.

Serra J, Collado A, Solà R, Antonelli F, Torres X, Salgueiro M, Quiles C, Bostock H. Hyperexcitable C nociceptors in fibromyalgia. Ann Neurol. 2014 Feb;75(2):196–208. PubMed PMID: 24243538.

Shang Y, Gurley K, Symons B, Long D, Srikuea R, Crofford LJ, Peterson CA, Yu G. Noninvasive optical characterization of muscle blood flow, oxygenation, and metabolism in women with fibromyalgia. Arthritis Res Ther. 2012 Nov 1;14(6):R236. PubMed PMID: 23116302.

Spaeth M, Fischer P, Langner C, Pongratz D. Increase of collagen IV in skeletal muscle of fibromyalgia patients. J Musculoskelet Pain 2005;12(9S):67.

Chapter 7. Rest: Taming the Hyperactive Stress Response

Bagis S, Karabiber M, As I, Tamer L, Erdogan C, Atalay A. Is magnesium citrate treatment effective on pain, clinical parameters and functional status in patients with fibromyalgia? Rheumatol Int. 2013 Jan;33(1):167–72. PubMed PMID: 22271372.

Cork RC, Wood P, Ming C, et al. The effect of cranial electrotherapy stimulation (CES) on pain associated with fibromyalgia. Internet J Anesthesiol 2004;8(2).

Cottingham JT, Porges SW, Richmond K. Shifts in pelvic inclination angle and parasympathetic tone produced by Rolfing soft tissue manipulation. Phys Ther. 1988 Sep;68(9):1364–70. PubMed PMID: 3420170.

Eisinger J, Plantamura A, Marie PA, Ayavou T. Selenium and magnesium status in fibromyalgia. Magnes Res. 1994 Dec; 7(3–4):285–88. PubMed PMID: 7786692.

Feinberg DA, Mark AS. Human brain motion and cerebrospinal fluid circulation demonstrated with MR velocity imaging. Radiology. 1987 Jun;163(3):793–99. PubMed PMID: 3575734.

Haker E, Egekvist H, Bjerring P. Effect of sensory stimulation (acupuncture) on sympathetic and parasympathetic activities in healthy subjects. J Auton Nerv Syst. 2000 Feb 14;79(1): 52–59. PubMed PMID: 10683506.

Imai K, Ariga H, Takahashi T. Electroacupuncture improves imbalance of autonomic function under restraint stress in conscious rats. Am J Chin Med. 2009;37(1):45–55. PubMed PMID: 19222111.

Kim YS, Kim KM, Lee DJ, Kim BT, Park SB, Cho DY, Suh CH, Kim HA, Park RW, Joo NS. Women with fibromyalgia have lower levels of calcium, magnesium, iron and manganese in hair mineral analysis. J Korean Med Sci. 2011 Oct;26(10): 1253–57. PubMed PMID: 22022174.

Lichtbroun AS, Raicer MM, Smith RB. The treatment of fibromyalgia with cranial electrotherapy stimulation. J Clin Rheumatol. 2001 Apr;7(2):72–78; discussion 78. PubMed PMID: 17039098.

Sakai S, Hori E, Umeno K, Kitabayashi N, Ono T, Nishijo H. Specific acupuncture sensation correlates with EEGs and autonomic changes in human subjects. Auton Neurosci. 2007 May 30;133(2):158–69. PubMed PMID: 17321222.

Tanaka S, Ito T. Histochemical demonstration of adrenergic fibers in the fascia periosteum and retinaculum. Clin Orthop Relat Res. 1977 Jul–Aug;(126):276–81. PubMed PMID: 598132.

van Dierendonck D, Nijenhuis JT. Flotation restricted environmental stimulation therapy (REST) as a stress-management tool: a meta-analysis. Psychol Health. 2005:20(3).

Chapter 8. Rest: Fixing Fibromyalgia Sleep

Branco J, Atalaia A, Paiva T. Sleep cycles and alpha-delta sleep in fibromyalgia syndrome. J Rheumatol. 1994 Jun;21(6):1113–17. PubMed PMID: 7932424.

Cho YW, Allen RP, Earley CJ. Lower molecular weight intravenous iron dextran for restless legs syndrome. Sleep Med. 2013 Mar;14(3):274–77. PubMed PMID: 23333678.

Davis, JL. Living with chronic fatigue. WebMD. No date. http://www.webmd.com/fibromyalgia/features/living-with-fibromyalgia-and-chronic-fatigue.

Dimsdale JE, Norman D, DeJardin D, Wallace MS. The effect of opioids on sleep architecture. J Clin Sleep Med. 2007 Feb 15;3(1):33–36. PubMed PMID: 17557450.

Feige B, Gann H, Brueck R, Hornyak M, Litsch S, Hohagen F, Riemann D. Effects of alcohol on polysomnographically recorded sleep in healthy subjects. Alcohol Clin Exp Res. 2006 Sep;30(9):1527–37. PubMed PMID: 16930215.

Gambacciani M, Ciaponi M, Cappagli B, Monteleone P, Benussi C, Bevilacqua G, Vacca F, Genazzani AR. Effects of low-dose, continuous combined hormone replacement therapy on sleep in symptomatic postmenopausal women. Maturitas. 2005 Feb 14;50(2):91–97. PubMed PMID: 15653005.

Gold AR, Dipalo F, Gold MS, Broderick J. Inspiratory airflow dynamics during sleep in women with fibromyalgia. Sleep. 2004 May 1;27(3):459–66. PubMed PMID: 15164899.

Hindmarch I, Dawson J, Stanley N. A double-blind study in healthy voluntcers to assess the effects on sleep of pregabalin compared with alprazolam and placebo. Sleep. 2005 Feb 1;28(2):187–93. PubMed PMID: 16171242.

Kooh M, Martínez-Lavín M, Meza S, Martín-del-Campo A, Hermosillo AG, Pineda C, Nava A, Amigo MC, Drucker-Colín R. Simultaneous heart rate variability and polysomnographic analyses in fibromyalgia. Clin Exp Rheumatol. 2003 Jul–Aug;21(4):529–30. PubMed PMID: 1294271.

May KP, West SG, Baker MR, Everett DW. Sleep apnea in male patients with the fibromyalgia syndrome. Am J Med. 1993 May;94(5):505–8. PubMed PMID: 8498395.

Moldofsky H. The significance of the sleeping-waking brain for the understanding of widespread musculoskeletal pain and fatigue in fibromyalgia syndrome and allied syndromes. Joint Bone Spine. 2008 Jul;75(4):397–402. PubMed PMID: 1845653.

Moldofsky H, Scarisbrick P, England R, Smythe H. Musculoskeletal symptoms and non-REM sleep disturbance in patients with "fibrositis syndrome" and healthy subjects. Psychosom Med. 1975 Jul–Aug;37(4):341–51. PubMed PMID: 169541.

Rosenfeld VW, Rutledge DN, Stern JM. Polysomnography with quantitative EEG in patients with and without fibromyalgia. J Clin Neurophysiol. 2015 Apr;32(2):164–70. PubMed PMID: 25233248.

Shah MA, Feinberg S, Krishnan E. Sleep-disordered breathing among women with fibromyalgia syndrome. J Clin Rheumatol. 2006 Dec;12(6):277–81. PubMed PMID: 17149057.

Shaw IR, Lavigne G, Mayer P, Choinière M. Acute intravenous administration of morphine perturbs sleep architecture in healthy pain-free young adults: a preliminary study. Sleep. 2005 Jun 1;28(6):677–82 PubMed PMID: 16477954.

Staud R. Sodium oxybate for the treatment of fibromyalgia. Expert Opin Pharmacother. 2011 Aug;12(11):1789–98. PubMed PMID: 21679091.

Viola-Saltzman M, Watson NF, Bogart A, Goldberg J, Buchwald D. High prevalence of restless legs syndrome among patients with fibromyalgia: a controlled cross-sectional study. J Clin Sleep Med. 2010 Oct 15;6(5):423–27. PubMed PMID: 20957840.

Xie L, Kang H, Xu Q, Chen MJ, Liao Y, Thiyagarajan M, O'Donnell J, Christensen DJ, Nicholson C, Iliff JJ, Takano T, Deane R, Nedergaard M. Sleep drives metabolite clearance from the adult brain. Science. 2013 Oct 18;342(6156):373–77. PubMed PMID: 24136970.

Chapter 9. Rest: Medications to Increase Deep Sleep

Billioti de Gage S, Bégaud B, Bazin F, Verdoux H, Dartigues JF, Pérès K, Kurth T, Pariente A. Benzodiazepine use and risk of dementia: prospective population based study. Brit Med J. 2012 Sep 27;345:e6231. PubMed PMID: 23045258.

Billioti de Gage S, Moride Y, Ducruet T, Kurth T, Verdoux H, Tournier M, Pariente A, Bégaud B. Benzodiazepine use and risk of Alzheimer's disease: case-control study. Brit Med J. 2014 Sep 9;349:g5205. PubMed PMID: 25208536.

Boehnlein JK, Kinzie JD. Pharmacologic reduction of CNS noradrenergic activity in PTSD: the case for clonidine and prazosin. J Psychiatr Pract. 2007 Mar;13(2):72–78. PubMed PMID: 17414682.

Brown MA, Guilleminault C. A review of sodium oxybate and baclofen in the treatment of sleep disorders. Curr Pharm Des. 2011;17(15):1430–35. PubMed PMID: 21476957.

Calandre EP, Rico-Villademoros F. The role of antipsychotics in the management of fibromyalgia. CNS Drugs. 2012 Feb 1; 26(2):135–53. PubMed PMID: 22296316.

Dimpfel W, Suter A. Sleep improving effects of a single dose administration of a valerian/hops fluid extract—a double blind, randomized, placebo-controlled sleep-EEG study in a parallel design using electrohypnograms. Eur J Med Res. 2008 May 26; 13(5):200–204. PubMed PMID: 18559301.

Drewes AM, Andreasen A, Jennum P, Nielsen KD. Zopiclone in the treatment of sleep abnormalities in fibromyalgia. Scand J Rheumatol. 1991;20(4):288–93. PubMed PMID: 1925417.

FDA (Food and Drug Administration). FDA Drug Safety Communication: Risk of next-morning impairment after use of insomnia drugs; FDA requires lower recommended doses for certain drugs containing zolpidem (Ambien, Ambien CR, Edluar, and Zolpimist). 2013 Jan 10. http://www.fda.gov/Drugs /DrugSafety/ucm334033.htm.

Feinberg I, Jones R, Walker JM, Cavness C, March J. Effects of high dosage delta-9-tetrahydrocannabinol on sleep patterns in man. Clin Pharmacol Ther. 1975 Apr;17(4):458–66. PubMed PMID: 164314.

Foldvary-Schaefer N, De Leon Sanchez I, Karafa M, Mascha E, Dinner D, Morris HH. Gabapentin increases slow-wave sleep in normal adults. Epilepsia. 2002 Dec;43(12):1493–97. PubMed PMID: 12460250.

Grönblad M, Nykänen J, Konttinen Y, Järvinen E, Helve T. Effect of zopiclone on sleep quality, morning stiffness, widespread tenderness and pain and general discomfort in primary fibromyalgia patients. A double-blind randomized trial. Clin Rheumatol. 1993 Jun;12(2):186–91. PubMed PMID: 8358976.

Held K, Antonijevic IA, Künzel H, Uhr M, Wetter TC, Golly IC, Steiger A, Murck H. Oral Mg(2+) supplementation reverses age-related neuroendocrine and sleep EEG changes in humans. Pharmacopsychiatry. 2002 Jul;35(4):135–43. PubMed PMID: 12163983.

Hidalgo J, Rico-Villademoros F, Calandre EP. An open-label study of quetiapine in the treatment of fibromyalgia. Prog Neuropsychopharmacol Biol Psychiatry. 2007 Jan 30;31(1):71–77. PubMed PMID: 16889882.

Hindmarch I, Dawson J, Stanley N. A double-blind study in healthy volunteers to assess the effects on sleep of pregabalin compared with alprazolam and placebo. Sleep. 2005 Feb;28(2): 187–93. PubMed PMID: 16171242.

Huang YS, Guilleminault C. Narcolepsy: action of two gamma-aminobutyric acid type B agonists, baclofen and sodium oxybate. Pediatr Neurol. 2009 Jul;41(1):9–16. PubMed PMID: 19520267.

Hunt GE, O'Sullivan BT, Johnson GF, Smythe GA. Growth hormone and cortisol secretion after oral clonidine in healthy adults. Psychoneuroendocrinology. 1986;11(3):317–25. PubMed PMID: 3786637.

Mathias S, Wetter TC, Steiger A, Lancel M. The GABA uptake inhibitor tiagabine promotes slow wave sleep in normal elderly subjects. Neurobiol Aging. 2001 Mar–Apr;22(2):247–53. PubMed PMID: 11182474.

Mendelson WB. A review of the evidence for the efficacy and safety of trazodone in insomnia. J Clin Psychiatry. 2005 Apr;66(4):469–76. PubMed PMID: 1581678.

Moldofsky H, Lue FA, Mously C, Roth-Schechter B, Reynolds WJ. The effect of zolpidem in patients with fibromyalgia: a dose ranging, double blind, placebo controlled, modified crossover study. J Rheumatol. 1996 Mar;23(3):529–33. PubMed PMID: 8832997.

Moldofsky H, Harris HW, Archambault WT, Kwong T, Lederman S. Effects of bedtime very low dose cyclobenzaprine on symptoms and sleep physiology in patients with fibromyalgia syndrome: a double-blind randomized placebo-controlled study. J Rheumatol. 2011 Dec;38(12):2653–63. PubMed PMID: 21885490.

Roth T, Lankford DA, Bhadra P, Whalen E, Resnick EM. Effect of pregabalin on sleep in patients with fibromyalgia and sleep maintenance disturbance: a randomized, placebo-controlled, 2-way crossover polysomnography study. Arthritis Care Res (Hoboken). 2012 Apr;64(4):597–606. PubMed PMID: 22232085.

Schittecatte M, Dumont F, Machowski R, Cornil C, Lavergne F, Wilmotte J. Effects of mirtazapine on sleep polygraphic variables in major depression. Neuropsychobiology. 2002;46(4): 197–201. PubMed PMID: 12566938.

Staud R. Sodium oxybate for the treatment of fibromyalgia. Expert Opin Pharmacother. 2011 Aug;12(11):1789–98. PubMed PMID: 21679091.

Stoschitzky K, Sakotnik A, Lercher P, Zweiker R, Maier R, Liebmann P, Lindner W. Influence of beta-blockers on melatonin release. Eur J Clin Pharmacol. 1999 Apr;55(2):111–15. PubMed PMID: 10335905.

Walsh JK, Perlis M, Rosenthal M, Krystal A, Jiang J, Roth T. Tiagabine increases slow-wave sleep in a dose-dependent fashion without affecting traditional efficacy measures in adults with primary insomnia. J Clin Sleep Med. 2006 Jan 15;2(1): 35–41. PubMed PMID: 17557435.

Walsh JK, Randazzo AC, Stone K, Eisenstein R, Feren SD, Kajy S, Dickey P, Roehrs T, Roth T, Schweitzer PK. Tiagabine is associated with sustained attention during sleep restriction: evidence for the value of slow-wave sleep enhancement? Sleep. 2006 Apr;29(4):433–43. PubMed PMID: 16676776.

Ware MA, Fitzcharles MA, Joseph L, Shir Y. The effects of nabilone on sleep in fibromyalgia: results of a randomized controlled trial. Anesth Analg. 2010 Feb 1;110(2):604–10. PubMed PMID: 20007734.

Yeephu S, Suthisisang C, Suttiruksa S, Prateepavanich P, Limampai P, Russell IJ. Efficacy and safety of mirtazapine in fibromyalgia syndrome patients: a randomized placebo-controlled pilot study. Ann Pharmacother. 2013 Jul–Aug;47 (7–8):921–32. PubMed PMID: 23737510.

Chapter 10. Repair: Digestion

Bjarnason I, MacPherson A, Hollander D. Intestinal permeability: an overview. Gastroenterology. 1995 May;108(5): 1566–81. PubMed PMID: 7729650.

Goebel A, Buhner S, Schedel R, Lochs H, Sprotte G. Altered intestinal permeability in patients with primary fibromyalgia and in patients with complex regional pain syndrome. Rheumatology (Oxford). 2008 Aug;47(8):1223–27. PubMed PMID: 18540025.

Meddings JB, Swain MG. Environmental stress-induced gastrointestinal permeability is mediated by endogenous glucocorticoids in the rat. Gastroenterology. 2000 Oct;119(4): 1019–28. PubMed PMID: 11040188.

Mennigen R, Bruewer M. Effect of probiotics on intestinal barrier function. Ann N Y Acad Sci. 2009 May;1165:183–89. PubMed PMID: 19538305.

Pali-Schöll I, Herzog R, Wallmann J, Szalai K, Brunner R, Lukschal A, Karagiannis P, Diesner SC, Jensen-Jarolim E. Antacids and dietary supplements with an influence on the gastric pH increase the risk for food sensitization. Clin Exp Allergy. 2010 Jul;40(7):1091–98. PubMed PMID: 20214670.

Pyleris E, Giamarellos-Bourboulis EJ, Tzivras D, Koussoulas V, Barbatzas C, Pimentel M. The prevalence of overgrowth by aerobic bacteria in the small intestine by small bowel culture: relationship with irritable bowel syndrome. Dig Dis Sci. 2012 May;57(5):1321–29. PubMed PMID: 22262197.

Quan ZF, Yang C, Li N, Li JS. Effect of glutamine on change in early postoperative intestinal permeability and its relation to systemic inflammatory response. World J Gastroenterol. 2004 Jul 1;10(13):1992–94. PubMed PMID: 15222054.

Quigley EM, Quera R. Small intestinal bacterial overgrowth: roles of antibiotics, prebiotics, and probiotics. Gastroenterology. 2006 Feb;130(2 Suppl 1):S78–90. PubMed PMID: 16473077.

Rapin JR, Wiernsperger N. Possible links between intestinal permeability and food processing: A potential therapeutic niche for glutamine. Clinics (São Paulo). 2010 Jun;65(6):635–43. PubMed PMID: 20613941.

Ukena SN, Singh A, Dringenberg U, Engelhardt R, Seidler U, Hansen W, Bleich A, Bruder D, Franzke A, Rogler G, Suerbaum S, Buer J, Gunzer F, Westendorf AM. Probiotic Escherichia coli Nissle 1917 inhibits leaky gut by enhancing mucosal integrity. PLoS One. 2007 Dec 12;2(12):c1308. PubMed PMID: 18074031.

Untersmayr E, Jensen-Jarolim E. The role of protein digestibility and antacids on food allergy outcomes. J Allergy Clin Immunol. 2008 Jun;121(6):1301–8. PubMed PMID: 18539189.

Veale D, Kavanagh G, Fielding JF, Fitzgerald O. Primary fibromyalgia and the irritable bowel syndrome: different expressions of a common pathogenetic process. Br J Rheumatol. 1991 Jun;30(3):220–22. PubMed PMID: 2049586.

Xu CL, Sun R, Qiao XJ, Xu CC, Shang XY, Niu WN. Protective effect of glutamine on intestinal injury and bacterial community in rats exposed to hypobaric hypoxia environment. World J Gastroenterol. 2014 Apr 28;20(16):4662–74. PubMed PMID: 24782618.

Yoon JS, Sohn W, Lee OY, Lee SP, Lee KN, Jun DW, Lee HL, Yoon BC, Choi HS, Chung WS, Seo JG. Effect of multispecies probiotics on irritable bowel syndrome: a randomized, double-blind, placebo-controlled trial. J Gastroenterol Hepatol. 2014 Jan;29(1):52–59. PubMed PMID: 23829297.

Chapter 11. Repair: Therapeutic Movement

Clark RA, Bryant AL, Pua Y, McCrory P, Bennell K, Hunt M. Validity and reliability of the Nintendo Wii Balance Board for assessment of standing balance. Gait Posture. 2010 Mar;31(3):307–10. PubMed PMID: 20005112.

Furlan R, Colombo S, Perego F, Atzeni F, Diana A, Barbic F, Porta A, Pace F, Malliani A, Sarzi-Puttini P. Abnormalities of cardiovascular neural control and reduced orthostatic tolerance in patients with primary fibromyalgia. J Rheumatol. 2005 Sep;32(9):1787–93. PubMed PMID: 16142879.

Gowans SE, deHueck A. Pool exercise for individuals with fibromyalgia. Curr Opin Rheumatol. 2007 Mar;19(2):168–73. PubMed PMID: 17278933.

Jones KD, Horak FB, Winters-Stone K, Irvine JM, Bennett RM. Fibromyalgia is associated with impaired balance and falls. J Clin Rheumatol. 2009 Feb;15(1):16–21. PubMed PMID: 19125137.

Jones KD, Liptan GL. Exercise interventions in fibromyalgia: clinical applications from the evidence. Rheum Dis Clin North Am. 2009 May;35(2):373–91. PubMed PMID: 19647149.

Nitz JC, Kuys S, Isles R, Fu S. Is the Wii Fit a new-generation tool for improving balance, health and well-being? A pilot study. Climacteric. 2010 Oct;13(5)487–91. PubMed PMID: 19905991.

Chapter 12. Repair: Unsticking the Fascia

Affaitati G, Costantini R, Fabrizio A, Lapenna D, Tafuri E, Giamberardino MA. Effects of treatment of peripheral pain generators in fibromyalgia patients. Eur J Pain. 2011 Jan;15(1): 61–69. PubMed PMID: 20889359.

Alonso-Blanco C, Fernández-de-las-Peñas C, Morales-Cabezas M, Zarco-Moreno P, Ge HY, Florez-García M. Multiple active myofascial trigger points reproduce the overall spontaneous pain pattern in women with fibromyalgia and are related to widespread mechanical hypersensitivity. Clin J Pain. 2011 Jun;27(5):405–13. PubMed PMID: 21368661.

Bonica JJ. The management of pain. Philadelphia: Lea & Febinger, 1990.

Cao TV, Hicks MR, Zein-Hammoud M, Standley PR. Duration and magnitude of myofascial release in 3-dimensional bioengineered tendons: effects on wound healing. J Am Osteopath Assoc. 2015 Feb;115(2):72–82. PubMed PMID: 25637613.

Castro-Sánchez AM, Matarán-Peñarrocha GA, Arroyo-Morales M, Saavedra-Hernández M, Fernández-Sola C, Moreno-Lorenzo C. Effects of myofascial release techniques on pain, physical function, and postural stability in patients with fibromyalgia: a randomized controlled trial. Clin Rehabil. 2011 Sep;25(9):800–813. PubMed PMID: 21673013.

Castro-Sánchez AM, Matarán-Peñarrocha GA, Granero-Molina J, Aguilera-Manrique G, Quesada-Rubio JM, Moreno-Lorenzo C. Benefits of massage–myofascial release therapy on pain, anxiety, quality of sleep, depression, and quality of life in patients with fibromyalgia. Evid Based Complement Alternat Med. 2011. PubMed PMID: 21234327.

Cheng N, Van Hoof H, Bockx E, Hoogmartens MJ, Mulier JC, De Dijcker FJ, Sansen WM, De Loecker W. The effects of electric currents on ATP generation, protein synthesis, and membrane transport of rat skin. Clin Orthop Relat Res. 1982 Nov–Dec;(171):264–72. PubMed PMID: 7140077.

Cottingham JT, Porges SW, Richmond K. Shifts in pelvic inclination angle and parasympathetic tone produced by Rolfing soft tissue manipulation. Phys Ther. 1988 Sep;68(9):1364–70. PubMed PMID: 3420170.

Gowers WR. Lumbago: its lessons and analogues. Br Med J. 1904 Jan 16;1(2246):117–21. PubMed PMID: 20761312.

Grimm D. Biomedical research. Cell biology meets Rolfing. Science. 2007 Nov 23;318(5854):1234–35. PubMed PMID: 18033859.

Hong CZ. Lidocaine injection versus dry needling to myofascial trigger point. The importance of the local twitch response. Am J Phys Med Rehabil. 1994 Jul–Aug;73(4):256–63. PubMed PMID: 8043247.

Hong CZ, Hsueh TC. Difference in pain relief after trigger point injections in myofascial pain patients with and without fibromyalgia. Arch Phys Med Rehabil. 1996 Nov;77(11): 1161–66. PubMed PMID: 8931529.

Kellgren JH. Referred pains from muscle. Brit Med J. 1938 Feb 12;1(4023):325–27. PubMed PMID: 20781237.

Liptan GL. Fascia: a missing link in our understanding of the pathology of fibromyalgia. J Bodyw Mov Ther. 2010 Jan;14(1):3–12. PubMed PMID: 20006283.

Liptan G, Mist S, Wright C, Arzt A, Jones KD. A pilot study of myofascial release therapy compared to Swedish massage in fibromyalgia. J Bodyw Mov Ther. 2013 Jul;17(3):365–70. PubMed PMID: 23768283.

McMakin C. Microcurrent treatment of myofascial pain in the head, neck and face. Top Clin Chiro. 1998 Mar;5(1):29–35.

———. Microcurrent therapy: a novel treatment method for chronic low back myofascial pain. J Bodyw Mov Ther. 2004; 8(2):143–53.

McMakin C, Gregory WM, Phillips TM. Cytokine changes with microcurrent treatment of fibromyalgia associated with cervical spine trauma. J Bodyw Mov Ther. 2005 Jul;9:169–76.

Staud R, Weyl EE, Bartley E, Price DD, Robinson ME. Analgesic and anti-hyperalgesic effects of muscle injections with lidocaine or saline in patients with fibromyalgia syndrome. Eur J Pain. 2014 Jul;18(6):803–12. PubMed PMID: 24193993.

Stecco C, Gagey O, Belloni A, Pozzuoli A, Porzionato A, Macchi V, Aldegheri R, De Caro R, Delmas V. Anatomy of the deep fascia of the upper limb. Second part: study of innervation. Morphologie. 2007 Mar;91(292):38–43. PubMed PMID: 17574469.

Stockman R. The causes and treatment of chronic rheumatism. Br Med J. 1904 Feb 27;1(2252):477–79. PubMed PMID: 20761381.

Chapter 13. Rebalance: Energy Production

Bachasson D, Guinot M, Wuyam B, Favre-Juvin A, Millet GY, Levy P, Verges S. Neuromuscular fatigue and exercise capacity in fibromyalgia syndrome. Arthritis Care Res (Hoboken). 2013 Mar;65(3):432–40. PubMed PMID: 22965792.

Binkley N, Gemar D, Engelke J, Gangnon R, Ramamurthy R, Krueger D, Drezner MK. Evaluation of ergocalciferol or cholecalciferol dosing, 1,600 IU daily or 50,000 IU monthly in older adults. J Clin Endocrinol Metab. 2011 Apr;96(4):981–88. PubMed PMID: 21289249.

Bouillon R, Verstuyf A. Vitamin D, mitochondria, and muscle. J Clin Endocrinol Metab. 2013 Mar;98(3):961–63. PubMed PMID: 23472232.

Cordero MD, Alcocer-Gómez E, de Miguel M, Culic O, Carrión AM, Alvarez-Suarez JM, Bullón P, Battino M, Fernández-Rodríguez A, Sánchez-Alcazar JA. Can coenzyme q10 improve clinical and molecular parameters in fibromyalgia? Antioxid Redox Signal. 2013 Oct 20;19(12):1356–61. PubMed PMID: 23458405.

Ding H, Zhang ZY, Zhang JW, Zhang Y. Role of mitochondrial quality control in exercise-induced health adaptation. Zhongguo Ying Yong Sheng Li Xue Za Zhi. 2013 Nov;29(6):543–53. PubMed PMID: 24654538.

Elenkov IJ, Wilder RL, Chrousos GP, Vizi ES. The sympathetic nerve—an integrative interface between two supersystems: the brain and the immune system. Pharmacol Rev. 2000 Dec;52(4):595–638. PubMed PMID: 11121511.

EWG (Environmental Working Group). EWG's 2015 shopper's guide to pesticides in produce. 2015. www.ewg.org/foodnews /summary.php.

Eyles DW, Smith S, Kinobe R, Hewison M, McGrath JJ. Distribution of the vitamin D receptor and 1 alpha-hydroxylase in human brain. J Chem. Neuroanat. 2005 Jan;29(1):21–30. PubMed PMID: 15589699.

Gerdle B, Forsgren MF, Bengtsson A, Leinhard OD, Sören B, Karlsson A, Brandejsky V, Lund E, Lundberg P. Decreased muscle concentrations of ATP and PCR in the quadriceps muscle of fibromyalgia patients—a 31P-MRS study. Eur J Pain. 2013 Sep;17(8):1205–15. PubMed PMID: 23364928.

Ghirlanda G, Oradei A, Manto A, Lippa S, Uccioli L, Caputo S, Greco AV, Littarru GP. Evidence of plasma CoQ10-lowering effect by HMG-CoA reductase inhibitors: a double-blind, placebo-controlled study. J Clin Pharmacol. 1993 Mar;33(3): 226–29. PubMed PMID: 8463436.

Heaney RP, Recker RR, Grote J, Horst RL, Armas LA. Vitamin D(3) is more potent than vitamin D(2) in humans. J Clin Endocrinol Metab. 2011 Mar;96(3):E447–52. PubMed PMID: 21177785.

Little JP, Safdar A, Benton CR, Wright DC. Skeletal muscle and beyond: the role of exercise as a mediator of systemic mitochondrial biogenesis. Appl Physiol Nutr Metab. 2011 Oct;36(5): 598–607. PubMed PMID: 21888528.

McClave SA, Snider HL. Dissecting the energy needs of the body. Curr Opin Clin Nutr Metab Care. 2001 Mar;4(2):143–47. PubMed PMID: 11224660.

Parikh S, Saneto R, Falk MJ, Anselm I, Cohen BH, Haas R, Medicine Society TM. A modern approach to the treatment of mitochondrial disease. Curr Treat Options Neurol. 2009 Nov;11(6):414–30. PubMed PMID: 19891905.

Park JH, Phothimat P, Oates CT, Hernanz-Schulman M, Olsen NJ. Use of P-31 magnetic resonance spectroscopy to detect metabolic abnormalities in muscles of patients with fibromyalgia. Arthritis Rheum. 1998 Mar;41(3):406–13. PubMed PMID: 9506567.

Rossini M, Di Munno O, Valentini G, Bianchi G, Biasi G, Cacace E, Malesci D, La Montagna G, Viapiana O, Adami S. Double-blind, multicenter trial comparing acetyl l-carnitine with placebo in the treatment of fibromyalgia patients. Clin Exp Rheumatol. 2007 Mar–Apr;25(2):182–88. PubMed PMID: 17543140.

Shang Y, Gurley K, Symons B, Long D, Srikuea R, Crofford LJ, Peterson CA, Yu G. Noninvasive optical characterization of muscle blood flow, oxygenation, and metabolism in women with fibromyalgia. Arthritis Res Ther. 2012 Nov 1;14(6):R236. PubMed PMID: 23116302.

Sinha A, Hollingsworth KG, Ball S, Cheetham T. Improving the vitamin D status of vitamin D deficient adults is associated with improved mitochondrial oxidative function in skeletal muscle. J Clin Endocrinol Metab. 2013 Mar;98(3):E509–13. PubMed PMID: 23393184.

Sundaram K, Panneerselvam KS. Oxidative stress and DNA single strand breaks in skeletal muscle of aged rats: role of carnitine and lipoicacid. Biogerontology. 2006 Apr;7(2):111–18. PubMed PMID: 16802114.

Teitelbaum JE, Johnson C, St Cyr J. The use of D-ribose in chronic fatigue syndrome and fibromyalgia: a pilot study. J Altern Complement Med. 2006 Nov;12(9):857–62. PubMed PMID: 17109576.

Chapter 14. Rebalance: Inflammation

Bazzichi L, Rossi A, Massimetti G, Giannaccini G, Giuliano T, De Feo F, Ciapparelli A, Dell'Osso L, Bombardieri S. Cytokine patterns in fibromyalgia and their correlation with clinical manifestations. Clin Exp Rheumatol. 2007 Mar–Apr;25(2): 225–30. PubMed PMID: 17543146.

Behm FG, Gavin IM, Karpenko O, Lindgren V, Gaitonde S, Gashkoff PA, Gillis BS. Unique immunologic patterns in fibromyalgia. BMC Clin Pathol. 2012 Dec 17;12:25. PubMed PMID: 23245186.

Belcaro G, Cesarone MR, Dugall M, Pellegrini L, Ledda A, Grossi MG, Togni S, Appendino G. Efficacy and safety of Meriva®, a curcumin-phosphatidylcholine complex, during extended administration in osteoarthritis patients. Altern Med Rev. 2010 Dec;15(4):337–44. PubMed PMID: 21194249.

Berger A, Crozier G, Bisogno T, Cavaliere P, Innis S, Di Marzo V. Anandamide and diet: inclusion of dietary arachidonate and docosahexaenoate leads to increased brain levels of the corresponding N-acylethanolamines in piglets. Proc Natl Acad Sci U S A. 2001 May 22;98(11):6402–6. PubMed PMID: 11353819.

Chandran B, Goel A. A randomized, pilot study to assess the efficacy and safety of curcumin in patients with active rheumatoid arthritis. Phytother Res. 2012 Nov;26(11):1719–25. PubMed PMID: 22407780.

Deodhar SD, Sethi R, Srimal RC. Preliminary study on antirheumatic activity of curcumin (diferuloyl methane). Indian J Med Res. 1980 Apr;71:632–34. PubMed PMID: 7390600.

Deuster PA, Jaffe RM. A novel treatment for fibromyalgia improves clinical outcomes in a community-based study. J Musculoskelet Pain. 1998;6(2):133–49.

Deutsch L. Evaluation of the effect of Neptune Krill Oil on chronic inflammation and arthritic symptoms. J Am Coll Nutr. 2007 Feb;26(1):39–48. PubMed PMID: 17353582.

Haack M, Sanchez E, Mullington JM. Elevated inflammatory markers in response to prolonged sleep restriction are associated with increased pain experience in healthy volunteers. Sleep. 2007 Sep 1;30(9):1145–52. PubMed PMID: 17910386.

Kremer JM, Lawrence DA, Petrillo GF, Litts LL, Mullaly PM, Rynes RI, Stocker RP, Parhami N, Greenstein NS, Fuchs BR, et al. Effects of high-dose fish oil on rheumatoid arthritis after stopping nonsteroidal antiinflammatory drugs. Clinical and immune correlates. Arthritis Rheum. 1995 Aug;38(8):1107–14. PubMed PMID: 7639807.

Lentz MJ, Landis CA, Rothermel J, Shaver JL. Effects of selective slow wave sleep disruption on musculoskeletal pain and fatigue in middle-aged women. J Rheumatol. 1999 Jul;26(7):1586–92. PubMed PMID: 10405949.

Ponikau JU, Sherris DA, Kern EB, Homburger HA, Frigas E, Gaffey TA, Roberts GD. The diagnosis and incidence of aller-

gic fungal sinusitis. Mayo Clin Proc. 1999 Sep;74(9):877–84. PubMed PMID: 10488788.

Ruggiero C, Lattanzio F, Lauretani F, Gasperini B, Andres-Lacueva C, Cherubini A. Omega-3 polyunsaturated fatty acids and immune-mediated diseases: inflammatory bowel disease and rheumatoid arthritis. Curr Pharm Des. 2009;15(36):4135–48. PubMed PMID: 20041815.

Sapone A, Bai JC, Ciacci C, Dolinsek J, Green PH, Hadjivassiliou M, Kaukinen K, Rostami K, Sanders DS, Schumann M, Ullrich R, Villalta D, Volta U, Catassi C, Fasano A. Spectrum of gluten-related disorders: consensus on new nomenclature and classification. BMC Med. 2012 Feb 7;10:13. PubMed PMID: 22313950.

Simopoulos AP. Omega-3 fatty acids in inflammation and autoimmune diseases. J Am Coll Nutr. 2002 Dec;21(6):495–505. PubMed PMID: 12480795.

Smith JD, Terpening CM, Schmidt SO, Gums JG. Relief of fibromyalgia symptoms following discontinuation of dietary excitotoxins. Ann Pharmacother. 2001 Jun;35(6):702–6. PubMed PMID: 11408989.

Sturgill J, McGee E, Menzies V. Unique cytokine signature in the plasma of patients with fibromyalgia. J Immunol Res. 2014;2014:938576. PubMed PMID: 24741634.

Taylor MJ, Ponikau JU, Sherris DA, Kern EB, Gaffey TA, Kephart G, Kita H. Detection of fungal organisms in eosinophilic mucin using a fluorescein-labeled chitin-specific binding protein. Otolaryngol Head Neck Surg. 2002 Nov;127(5):377–83. PubMed PMID: 12447230.

Tyndall DA, Rathore S. Cone-beam CT diagnostic applications: caries, periodontal bone assessment, and endodontic ap-

plications. Dent Clin North Am. 2008 Oct;52(4):825–41, vii. PubMed PMID: 18805231.

Wang H, Moser M, Schiltenwolf M, Buchner M. Circulating cytokine levels compared to pain in patients with fibromyalgia, a prospective longitudinal study over six months. J Rheumatol. 2008 Jul;35(7):1366–70. PubMed PMID: 18528959.

Chapter 15. Rebalance: Adrenal Hormones

Aardal E, Holm AC. Cortisol in saliva—reference ranges and relation to cortisol in serum. Eur J Clin Chem Clin Biochem. 1995 Dec;33(12):927–32. PubMed PMID: 8845424.

Bhattacharya SK, Muruganandam AV. Adaptogenic activity of Withania somnifera: an experimental study using a rat model of chronic stress. Pharmacol Biochem Behav. 2003 Jun;75(3): 547–55. PubMed PMID: 12895672.

Blockmans D, Persoons P, Van Houdenhove B, Lejeune M, Bobbaers H. Combination therapy with hydrocortisone and fludrocortisone does not improve symptoms in chronic fatigue syndrome: a randomized, placebo-controlled, double-blind, crossover study. Am J Med. 2003 Jun 15;114(9):736–41. PubMed PMID: 12829200.

Chandrasekhar K, Kapoor J, Anishetty S. A prospective, randomized double-blind, placebo-controlled study of safety and efficacy of a high-concentration full-spectrum extract of ashwagandha root in reducing stress and anxiety in adults. Indian J Psychol Med. 2012 Jul;34(3):255–62. PubMed PMID: 23439798.

Cleare AJ, Heap E, Malhi GS, Wessely S, O'Keane V, Miell J. Low-dose hydrocortisone in chronic fatigue syndrome: a ran-

domised crossover trial. Lancet. 1999 Feb 6;353(9151):455–58. PubMed PMID: 9989716.

Hellhammer J, Vogt D, Franz N, Freitas U, Rutenberg D. A soy-based phosphatidylserine/phosphatidic acid complex (PAS) normalizes the stress reactivity of hypothalamus-pituitary-adrenal-axis in chronically stressed male subjects: a randomized, placebo-controlled study. Lipids Health Dis. 2014 Jul 31;13(1):121. PubMed PMID: 25081826.

Ishaque S, Shamseer L, Bukutu C, Vohra S. Rhodiola rosea for physical and mental fatigue: a systematic review. BMC Complement Altern Med. 2012 May 29;12:70. PubMed PMID: 22643043.

Mahdi AA, Fatima G, Das SK, Verma NS. Abnormality of circadian rhythm of serum melatonin and other biochemical parameters in fibromyalgia syndrome. Indian J Biochem Biophys. 2011 Apr;48(2):82–87. PubMed PMID: 21682138.

McKenzie R, O'Fallon A, Dale J, Demitrack M, Sharma G, Deloria M, Garcia-Borreguero D, Blackwelder W, Straus SE. Low-dose hydrocortisone for treatment of chronic fatigue syndrome: a randomized controlled trial. JAMA. 1998 Sep 23–30; 280(12): 1061–66. PubMed PMID: 9757853.

Merza Z. Chronic use of opioids and the endocrine system. Horm Metab Res. 2010 Aug;42(9):621–26. PubMed PMID: 20486065.

Monteleone P, Beinat L, Tanzillo C, Maj M, Kemali D. Effects of phosphatidylserine on the neuroendocrine response to physical stress in humans. Neuroendocrinology. 1990 Sep;52(3): 243–48. PubMed PMID: 2170852.

Monteleone P, Maj M, Beinat L, Natale M, Kemali D. Blunting by chronic phosphatidylserine administration of the stress-induced activation of the hypothalamo-pituitary-adrenal axis in healthy men. Eur J Clin Pharmacol. 1992;42(4):385–88. PubMed PMID: 1325348.

Müssig K, Knaus-Dittmann D, Schmidt H, Mörike K, Häring HU. Secondary adrenal failure and secondary amenorrhoea following hydromorphone treatment. Clin Endocrinol (Oxford). 2007 Apr;66(4):604–5. PubMed PMID: 17371484.

Olsson EM, von Schéele B, Panossian AG. A randomised, double-blind, placebo-controlled, parallel-group study of the standardised extract shr-5 of the roots of Rhodiola rosea in the treatment of subjects with stress-related fatigue. Planta Med. 2009 Feb;75(2):105–12. PubMed PMID: 19016404.

Oltmanns KM, Fehm HL, Peters A. Chronic fentanyl application induces adrenocortical insufficiency. J Intern Med. 2005 May;257(5):478–80. PubMed PMID: 15836666.

Panossian A, Hambardzumyan M, Hovhanissyan A, Wikman G. The adaptogens rhodiola and schizandra modify the response to immobilization stress in rabbits by suppressing the increase of phosphorylated stress-activated protein kinase, nitric oxide and cortisol. Drug Target Insights. 2007;2:39–54. PubMed PMID: 21901061.

Pullan PT, Watson FE, Seow SS, Rappeport W. Methadone-induced hypoadrenalism. Lancet. 1983 Mar 26;1(8326 Pt 1): 714. PubMed PMID: 6132074.

Reber SO, Birkeneder L, Veenema AH, Obermeier F, Falk W, Straub RH, Neumann ID. Adrenal insufficiency and colonic inflammation after a novel chronic psycho-social stress paradigm in mice: implications and mechanisms. Endocrinology. 2007 Feb;148(2):670–82. PubMed PMID: 17110427.

Riedel W, Layka H, Neeck G. Secretory pattern of GH, TSH, thyroid hormones, ACTH, cortisol, FSH, and LH in patients with fibromyalgia syndrome following systemic injection of the relevant hypothalamic-releasing hormones. Z Rheumatol. 1998;57 Suppl 2:81–87. PubMed PMID: 10025090.

Riva R, Mork PJ, Westgaard RH, Rø M, Lundberg U. Fibromyalgia syndrome is associated with hypocortisolism. Int J Behav Med. 2010 Sep;17(3):223–33. PubMed PMID: 20458566.

Starks MA, Starks SL, Kingsley M, Purpura M, Jäger R. The effects of phosphatidylserine on endocrine response to moderate intensity exercise. J Int Soc Sports Nutr. 2008 Jul 28;5:11. PubMed PMID:18662395.

Chapter 16. Rebalance: Thyroid and Sex Hormones

Bazzichi L, Rossi A, Giuliano T, De Feo F, Giacomelli C, Consensi A, Ciapparelli A, Consoli G, Dell'osso L, Bombardieri S. Association between thyroid autoimmunity and fibromyalgic disease severity. Clin Rheumatol. 2007 Dec;26(12):2115–20. PubMed PMID: 17487449.

Brill KT, Weltman AL, Gentili A, Patrie JT, Fryburg DA, Hanks JB, Urban RJ, Veldhuis JD. Single and combined effects of growth hormone and testosterone administration on measures of body composition, physical performance, mood, sexual function, bone turnover, and muscle gene expression in healthy older men. J Clin Endocrinol Metab. 2002 Dec;87(12):5649–57. PubMed PMID: 12466367.

Daniell HW. Hypogonadism in men consuming sustained-action oral opioids. J Pain. 2002 Oct;3(5):377–84. PubMed PMID: 14622741.

Gambacciani M, Ciaponi M, Cappagli B, Monteleone P, Benussi C, Bevilacqua G, Vacca F, Genazzani AR. Effects of low-dose, continuous combined hormone replacement therapy on sleep in symptomatic postmenopausal women. Maturitas. 2005 Feb 14;50(2):91–97. PubMed PMID: 15653005.

Hoang TD, Olsen CH, Mai VQ, Clyde PW, Shakir MK. Desiccated thyroid extract compared with levothyroxine in the treatment of hypothyroidism: a randomized, double-blind, crossover study. J Clin Endocrinol Metab. 2013 May;98(5):1982–90. PubMed PMID: 23539727.

Holtorf K. The bioidentical hormone debate: are bioidentical hormones (estradiol, estriol, and progesterone) safer or more efficacious than commonly used synthetic versions in hormone replacement therapy? Postgrad Med. 2009 Jan;121(1):73–85. PubMed PMID: 19179815.

Hough JP, Papacosta E, Wraith E, Gleeson M. Plasma and salivary steroid hormone responses of men to high-intensity cycling and resistance exercise. J Strength Cond Res. 2011 Jan;25(1):23–31. PubMed PMID: 21157386.

Kralik A, Eder K, Kirchgessner M. Influence of zinc and selenium deficiency on parameters relating to thyroid hormone metabolism. Horm Metab Res. 1996 May;28(5):223–26. PubMed PMID: 8738110.

L'hermite M, Simoncini T, Fuller S, Genazzani AR. Could transdermal estradiol + progesterone be a safer postmenopausal HRT? A review. Maturitas. 2008 Jul–Aug;60(3–4):185–201. PubMed PMID: 18775609.

Malkin CJ, Pugh PJ, Morris PD, Asif S, Jones TH, Channer KS. Low serum testosterone and increased mortality in men with coronary heart disease. Heart. 2010 Nov;96(22):1821–25. PubMed PMID: 20959649.

Miller WL. Steroid hormone synthesis in mitochondria. Mol Cell Endocrinol. 2013 Oct 15;379(1–2):62–73. PubMed PMID: 23628605.

Olivieri O, Girelli D, Stanzial AM, Rossi L, Bassi A, Corrocher R. Selenium, zinc, and thyroid hormones in healthy subjects: low T3/T4 ratio in the elderly is related to impaired selenium status. Biol Trace Elem Res. 1996 Jan;51(1):31–41. PubMed PMID: 8834378.

Pamuk ON, Cakir N. The variation in chronic widespread pain and other symptoms in fibromyalgia patients. The effects of menses and menopause. Clin Ex Rheumatol. 2005 Nov–Dec;23(6):778–82. PubMed PMID: 16396694.

Panicker V, Saravanan P, Vaidya B, Evans J, Hattersley AT, Frayling TM, Dayan CM. Common variation in the DIO2 gene predicts baseline psychological well-being and response to combination thyroxine plus triiodothyronine therapy in hypothyroid patients. J Clin Endocrinol Metab 2009;94:1623–29. PubMed PMID: 191900113.

Rhoden EL, Morgentaler A. Risks of testosterone-replacement therapy and recommendations for monitoring. N Engl J Med. 2004 Jan 29;350(5):482–92. Review. PubMed PMID: 14749457.

Riedel W, Layka H, Neeck G. Secretory pattern of GH, TSH, thyroid hormones, ACTH, cortisol, FSH, and LH in patients with fibromyalgia syndrome following systemic injection of the relevant hypothalamic-releasing hormones. Z Rheumatol. 1998;57 Suppl 2:81–87. PubMed PMID: 10025090.

Roddam AW, Allen NE, Appleby P, Key TJ. Endogenous sex hormones and prostate cancer: a collaborative analysis of 18 prospective studies. J Natl Cancer Inst. 2008 Feb 6;100(3): 170–83. PubMed PMID: 18230794.

Schwarz ER, Phan A, Willix RD Jr. Andropause and the development of cardiovascular disease presentation—more than an epi-phenomenon. J Geriatr Cardiol. 2011 Mar;8(1):35–43. PubMed PMID: 22783283.

Smith HS, Elliott JA. Opioid-induced androgen deficiency (OPIAD). Pain Physician. 2012 Jul;15(3 Suppl):ES145–56. PubMed PMID: 22786453.

Soy M, Guldiken S, Arikan E, Altun BU, Tugrul A. Frequency of rheumatic diseases in patients with autoimmune thyroid disease. Rheumatol Int. 2007 Apr;27(6):575–77. PubMed PMID: 17102943.

Stening KD, Eriksson O, Henriksson KG, Brynhildsen J, Lindh-Åstrand L, Berg G, Hammar M, Amandusson A, Blomqvist A. Hormonal replacement therapy does not affect self-estimated pain or experimental pain responses in post-menopausal women suffering from fibromyalgia: a double-blind, randomized, placebo-controlled trial. Rheumatology (Oxford). 2011 Mar;50(3):544–51. PubMed PMID: 21078629.

Traish AM, Saad F, Guay A. The dark side of testosterone deficiency: II. Type 2 diabetes and insulin resistance. J Androl. 2009 Jan–Feb;30(1):23–32. PubMed PMID: 18772488.

Tsigos C, Chrousos GP. Hypothalamic-pituitary-adrenal axis, neuroendocrine factors and stress. J Psychosom Res. 2002 Oct;53(4):865–71. PubMed PMID: 12377295.

Vigen R, O'Donnell CI, Barón AE, Grunwald GK, Maddox TM, Bradley SM, Barqawi A, Woning G, Wierman ME, Plomondon ME, Rumsfeld JS, Ho PM. Association of testosterone therapy with mortality, myocardial infarction, and stroke in men with low testosterone levels. JAMA. 2013 Nov 6;310(17):1829–36 PubMed PMID: 24193080.

Woods NF, Lentz MJ, Mitchell ES, Shaver J, Heitkemper M. Luteal phase ovarian steroids, stress arousal, premenses perceived stress, and premenstrual symptoms. Res Nurs Health. 1998 Apr;21(2):129–42. PubMed PMID: 9535405.

Xu L, Freeman G, Cowling BJ, Schooling CM. Testosterone therapy and cardiovascular events among men: a systematic review and meta-analysis of placebo-controlled randomized trials. BMC Med. 2013 Apr 18;11:108. PubMed PMID: 23597181.

Yoshikawa GT, Heymann RE, Helfenstein M Jr, Pollak DF. A comparison of quality of life, demographic and clinical characteristics of Brazilian men with fibromyalgia syndrome with male patients with depression. Rheumatol Int. 2010 Feb;30(4): 473–78. PubMed PMID: 19562343.

Zimmermann MB, Köhrle J. The impact of iron and selenium deficiencies on iodine and thyroid metabolism: biochemistry and relevance to public health. Thyroid. 2002 Oct;12(10): 867–78. PubMed PMID: 12487769.

Chapter 17. Rebalance: Mood

Arnold LM, Hudson JI, Hess EV, Ware AE, Fritz DA, Auchenbach MB, Starck LO, Keck PE Jr. Family study of fibromyalgia. Arthritis Rheum. 2004 Mar;50(3):944–52. PubMed PMID: 15022338.

Cloitre M. Effective psychotherapies for posttraumatic stress disorder: a review and critique. CNS Spectr. 2009 Jan;14(1 Suppl 1):32–43. PubMed PMID: 19169192.

Coppen A, Bailey J. Enhancement of the antidepressant action of fluoxetine by folic acid: a randomised, placebo controlled trial. J Affect Disord. 2000 Nov;60(2):121–30. PubMed PMID: 10967371.

Dodhia S, Hosanagar A, Fitzgerald DA, Labuschagne I, Wood AG, Nathan PJ, Phan KL. Modulation of resting-state amygdala-frontal functional connectivity by oxytocin in generalized social anxiety disorder. Neuropsychopharmacology. 2014 Aug; 39(9):2061–69. PubMed PMID: 24594871.

Dyck JB, Chung F. A comparison of propranolol and diazepam for preoperative anxiolysis. Can J Anaesth. 1991 Sep;38(6): 704–9. PubMed PMID: 1914053.

Godfrey PS, Toone BK, Carney MW, Flynn TG, Bottiglieri T, Laundy M, Chanarin I, Reynolds EH. Enhancement of recovery from psychiatric illness by methylfolate. Lancet. 1990 Aug 18;336(8712):392–95. PubMed PMID: 1974941.

Grachev ID, Fredrickson BE, Apkarian AV. Abnormal brain chemistry in chronic back pain: an in vivo proton magnetic resonance spectroscopy study. Pain. 2000 Dec 15;89(1):7–18. PubMed PMID: 11113288.

Gustin SM, Peck CC, Macey PM, Murray GM, Henderson LA. Unraveling the effects of plasticity and pain on personality. J Pain. 2013 Dec;14(12):1642–52. PubMed PMID: 24290444.

Ishaque S, Shamseer L, Bukutu C, Vohra S. Rhodiola rosea for physical and mental fatigue: a systematic review. BMC Complement Altern Med. 2012 May 29;12:70. PubMed PMID: 22643043.

Kelly CB, McDonnell AP, Johnston TG, Mulholland C, Cooper SJ, McMaster D, Evans A, Whitehead AS. The MTHFR C677T polymorphism is associated with depressive episodes in patients from Northern Ireland. J Psychopharmacol. 2004 Dec;18(4):567–71. PubMed PMID: 15582924.

Khadke VV, Khadke SV, Khare A. Oral propranolol—efficacy and comparison of two doses for peri-operative anxiolysis. J Indian Med Assoc. 2012 Jul;110(7):457–60. PubMed PMID: 23520670.

Kirsch P, Esslinger C, Chen Q, Mier D, Lis S, Siddhanti S, Gruppe H, Mattay VS, Gallhofer B, Meyer-Lindenberg A. Oxytocin modulates neural circuitry for social cognition and fear in humans. J Neurosci. 2005 Dec 7;25(49):11489–93. PubMed PMID: 16339042.

Krueger C, Hawkins K, Wong S, Enns MW, Minuk G, Rempel JD. Persistent pro-inflammatory cytokines following the initiation of pegylated IFN therapy in hepatitis C infection is associated with treatment-induced depression. J Viral Hepat. 2011 Jul;18(7):e284–91. PubMed PMID: 21143344.

Labuschagne I, Phan KL, Wood A, Angstadt M, Chua P, Heinrichs M, Stout JC, Nathan PJ. Oxytocin attenuates amygdala reactivity to fear in generalized social anxiety disorder. Neuropsychopharmacology. 2010 Nov;35(12):2403–13. PubMed PMID: 20720535.

Lavigne JE, Heckler C, Mathews JL, Palesh O, Kirshner JJ, Lord R, Jacobs A, Amos E, Morrow GR, Mustian K. A randomized, controlled, double-blinded clinical trial of gabapentin 300 versus 900 mg versus placebo for anxiety symptoms in breast cancer survivors. Breast Cancer Res Treat. 2012 Nov;136(2):479–86. PubMed PMID: 23053645.

Lewis SJ, Lawlor DA, Davey Smith G, Araya R, Timpson N, Day IN, Ebrahim S. The thermolabile variant of MTHFR is associated with depression in the British Women's Heart and Health Study and a meta-analysis. Mol Psychiatry. 2006 Apr; 11(4):352–60. PubMed PMID: 16402130.

Maes M, Mylle J, Delmeire L, Altamura C. Psychiatric morbidity and comorbidity following accidental man-made traumatic events: incidence and risk factors. Eur Arch Psychiatry Clin Neurosci. 2000;250(3):156–62. PubMed PMID: 10941992.

Miller AL. The methylation, neurotransmitter, and antioxidant connections between folate and depression. Altern Med Rev. 2008 Sep;13(3):216–26. Pubmed PMID: 18950248.

Oschman, JL. Energy medicine: the scientific basis. Edinburgh: Churchill Livingstone, 2000.

Passeri M, Cucinotta D, Abate G, Senin U, Ventura A, Stramba Badiale M, Diana R, La Greca P, Le Grazie C. Oral 5'-methyltetrahydrofolic acid in senile organic mental disorders with depression: results of a double-blind multicenter study. Aging (Milano). 1993 Feb;5(1):63–71. PubMed PMID: 8257478.

Seto A, Kusaka C, Nakazato S, Huang WR, Sato T, Hisamitsu T, Takeshige C. Detection of extraordinary large bio-magnetic field strength from human hand during external Qi emission. Acupunct Electrother Res. 1992;17(2):75–94. PubMed PMID: 1353653.

Taylor HR, Freeman MK, Cates ME. Prazosin for treatment of nightmares related to posttraumatic stress disorder. Am J Health Syst Pharm. 2008 Apr 15;65(8):716–22. PubMed PMID: 18387899.

Tsao CW, Lin YS, Chen CC, Bai CH, Wu SR. Cytokines and serotonin transporter in patients with major depression. Prog Neuropsychopharmacol Biol Psychiatry. 2006 Jul;30(5): 899–905. PubMed PMID: 16616982.

Walker EA, Keegan D, Gardner G, Sullivan M, Katon WJ, Bernstein D. Psychosocial factors in fibromyalgia compared with rheumatoid arthritis: I. Psychiatric diagnoses and functional disability. Psychosom Med. 1997 Nov–Dec;59(6):565–71. PubMed PMID: 9407573.

Zimmerman J. Laying-on-of-hands healing and therapeutic touch: a testable theory. BEMI Currents, Journal of the Bio-Electro-Magnetics Institute 1990;2:8–17.

Chapter 18. Reduce: Fatigue and Fibrofog

Abbott A. Gaming improves multitasking skills. Nature. 2013 Sep 5;501(7465):18. PubMed PMID: 24005397.

Etnier JL, Karper WB, Gapin JI, Barella LA, Chang YK, Murphy KJ. Exercise, fibromyalgia, and fibrofog: a pilot study. J Phys Act Health. 2009 Mar;6(2):239–46. PubMed PMID: 19420402.

Glass JM. Fibromyalgia and cognition. J Clin Psychiatry. 2008;69 Suppl 2:20–24. PubMed PMID: 18537459.

———. Review of cognitive dysfunction in fibromyalgia: a convergence on working memory and attentional control impairments. Rheum Dis Clin North Am. 2009 May;35(2):299–311. PubMed PMID: 19647144.

Glass JM, Williams DA, Fernandez-Sanchez ML, Kairys A, Barjola P, Heitzeg MM, Clauw DJ, Schmidt-Wilcke T. Executive function in chronic pain patients and healthy controls: different cortical activation during response inhibition in fibromyalgia. J Pain. 2011 Dec;12(12):1219–29. PubMed PMID: 21945593.

Greer BK, White JP, Arguello EM, Haymes EM. Branched-chain amino acid supplementation lowers perceived exertion but does not affect performance in untrained males. J Strength Cond Res. 2011 Feb;25(2):539–44. PubMed PMID: 20386134.

Greer BK, Woodard JL, White JP, Arguello EM, Haymes EM. Branched-chain amino acid supplementation and indicators of muscle damage after endurance exercise. Int J Sport Nutr Exerc Metab. 2007 Dec;17(6):595–607. PubMed PMID: 18156664.

Jedrziewski MK, Ewbank DC, Wang H, Trojanowski JQ. Exercise and cognition: results from the National Long Term Care Survey. Alzheimers Dement. 2010 Nov;6(6):448–55. PubMed PMID: 21044775.

Kobayashi S, Iwamoto M, Kon K, Waki H, Ando S, Tanaka Y. Acetyl-L-carnitine improves aged brain function. Geriatr Gerontol Int. 2010 Jul;10 Suppl 1:S99–106. PubMed PMID: 20590847.

Leavitt F, Katz RS. Distraction as a key determinant of impaired memory in patients with fibromyalgia. J Rheumatol. 2006 Jan;33(1):127–32. PubMed PMID: 16395760.

Liu J. The effects and mechanisms of mitochondrial nutrient alpha-lipoic acid on improving age-associated mitochondrial and cognitive dysfunction: an overview. Neurochem Res. 2008 Jan;33(1):194–203. PubMed PMID:17605107.

Munguía-Izquierdo D, Legaz-Arrese A. Exercise in warm water decreases pain and improves cognitive function in middle-aged women with fibromyalgia. Clin Exp Rheumatol. 2007 Nov–Dec;25(6):823–30. PubMed PMID: 18173915.

Orsucci D, Mancuso M, Ienco EC, LoGerfo A, Siciliano G. Targeting mitochondrial dysfunction and neurodegeneration by means of coenzyme Q10 and its analogues. Curr Med Chem. 2011;18(26):4053–64. PubMed PMID: 21824087.

Pachas WN. Modafinil for the treatment of fatigue of fibromyalgia. J Clin Rheumatol. 2003 Aug;9(4):282–85. PubMed PMID: 17041476.

Packer L, Tritschler HJ, Wessel K. Neuroprotection by the metabolic antioxidant alpha-lipoic acid. Free Radic Biol Med. 1997;22(1–2):359–78. PubMed PMID: 8958163.

Park DC, Glass JM, Minear M, Crofford LJ. Cognitive function in fibromyalgia patients. Arthritis Rheum. 2001 Sep;44(9): 2125–33. PubMed PMID: 11592377.

Schaefer C, Chandran A, Hufstader M, Baik R, McNett M, Goldenberg D, Gerwin R, Zlateva G. The comparative burden of mild, moderate and severe fibromyalgia: results from a cross-sectional survey in the United States. Health Qual Life Outcomes. 2011 Aug 22;9:71. PubMed PMID: 21859448.

Schaller JL, Behar D. Modafinil in fibromyalgia treatment. J Neuropsychiatry Clin Neurosci. 2001 Fall;13(4):530–31. PubMed PMID: 11748325.

Schmitt R, Capo T, Frazier H, Boren D. Cranial electrotherapy stimulation treatment of cognitive brain dysfunction in chemical dependence. J Clin Psychiatry. 1984 Feb;45(2):60–61, 62–63. PubMed PMID: 6363398.

Schwartz TL, Rayancha S, Rashid A, Chlebowksi S, Chilton M, Morell M. Modafinil treatment for fatigue associated with fibromyalgia. J Clin Rheumatol. 2007 Feb;13(1):52. PubMed PMID: 17278955.

Schwartz TL, Siddiqui UA, Raza S, Morell M. Armodafinil for fibromyalgia fatigue. Ann Pharmacother. 2010 Jul–Aug;44 (7–8):1347–48. PubMed PMID: 20551299.

Suchy J, Chan A, Shea TB. Dietary supplementation with a combination of alpha-lipoic acid, acetyl-L-carnitine, glycerophosphocoline, docosahexaenoic acid, and phosphatidylserine reduces oxidative damage to murine brain and improves cognitive performance. Nutr Res. 2009 Jan;29(1):70–74. PubMed PMID: 19185780.

Young JL, Redmond JC. Fibromyalgia, chronic fatigue, and adult attention deficit hyperactivity disorder in the adult: a case study. Psychopharmacol Bull. 2007;40(1):118–26. PubMed PMID: 17285103.

Chapter 19. Reduce: Pain Hypersensitivity

Ametov AS, Barinov A, Dyck PJ, Hermann R, Kozlova N, Litchy WJ, Low PA, Nehrdich D, Novosadova M, O'Brien PC, Reljanovic M, Samigullin R, Schuette K, Strokov I, Tritschler HJ, Wessel K, Yakhno N, Ziegler D; SYDNEY Trial Study Group. The sensory symptoms of diabetic polyneuropathy are improved with alpha-lipoic acid: the SYDNEY trial. Diabetes Care. 2003 Mar;26(3):770–76. PubMed PMID: 12610036.

Amin P, Sturrock ND. A pilot study of the beneficial effects of amantadine in the treatment of painful diabetic peripheral neuropathy. Diabet Med. 2003 Feb;20(2):114–18. PubMed PMID: 12581262.

Argoff CE. A review of the use of topical analgesics for myofascial pain. Curr Pain Headache Rep. 2002 Oct;6(5):375–78. PubMed PMID: 12207850.

Arnold LM, Goldenberg DL, Stanford SB, Lalonde JK, Sandhu HS, Keck PE Jr, Welge JA, Bishop F, Stanford KE, Hess EV, Hudson JI. Gabapentin in the treatment of fibromyalgia: a randomized, double-blind, placebo-controlled, multicenter trial. Arthritis Rheum. 2007 Apr;56(4):1336–44. PubMed PMID: 17393438.

Cagnie B, Coppieters I, Denecker S, Six J, Danneels L, Meeus M. Central sensitization in fibromyalgia? A systematic review on structural and functional brain MRI. Semin Arthritis Rheum. 2014 Aug;44(1):68–75. PubMed PMID: 24508406.

Campbell CM, Kipnes MS, Stouch BC, Brady KL, Kelly M, Schmidt WK, Petersen KL, Rowbotham MC, Campbell JN.

Randomized control trial of topical clonidine for treatment of painful diabetic neuropathy. Pain. 2012 Sep;153(9):1815–23. PubMed PMID: 22683276.

Challapalli V, Tremont-Lukats IW, McNicol ED, Lau J, Carr DB. Systemic administration of local anesthetic agents to relieve neuropathic pain. Cochrane Database Syst Rev. 2005 Oct 19;(4):CD003345. Review. PubMed PMID: 16235318.

Choi DK, Koppula S, Suk K. Inhibitors of microglial neurotoxicity: focus on natural products. Molecules. 2011 Jan 25;16(2):1021–43. PubMed PMID: 21350391.

Clauw DJ. Pharmacotherapy for patients with fibromyalgia. J Clin Psychiatry. 2008; 69 Suppl 2:25–29. PubMed PMID: 18537460.

de Mos M, Huygen FJ, Stricker BH, Dieleman JP, Sturkenboom MC. The association between ACE inhibitors and the complex regional pain syndrome: suggestions for a neuro-inflammatory pathogenesis of CRPS. Pain. 2009 Apr;142(3):218–24. PubMed PMID: 19195784.

Dominkus M, Nicolakis M, Kotz R, Wilkinson FE, Kaiser RR, Chlud K. Comparison of tissue and plasma levels of ibuprofen after oral and topical administration. Arzneimittelforschung. 1996 Dec;46(12):1138–43. PubMed PMID: 900678.

Finch PM, Knudsen L, Drummond PD. Reduction of allodynia in patients with complex regional pain syndrome: a double-blind placebo-controlled trial of topical ketamine. Pain. 2009 Nov;146(1–2):18–25. PubMed PMID: 19703730.

Gilliam WP, Burns JW, Gagnon C, Stanos S, Matsuura J, Beckman N. Strategic self-presentation may enhance effects of interdisciplinary chronic pain treatment. Health Psychol. 2013 Feb;32(2):156–63. PubMed PMID: 22888822.

Gracely RH, Geisser ME, Giesecke T, Grant MA, Petzke F, Williams DA, Clauw DJ. Pain catastrophizing and neural responses to pain among persons with fibromyalgia. Brain. 2004 Apr; 127(Pt 4):835–43. PubMed PMID: 14960499.

Heyneman CA, Lawless-Liday C, Wall GC. Oral versus topical NSAIDs in rheumatic diseases: a comparison. Drugs. 2000 Sep;60(3):555–74. PubMed PMID: 11030467.

Hoffman BM, Papas RK, Chatkoff DK, Kerns RD. Meta-analysis of psychological interventions for chronic low back pain. Health Psychol. 2007 Jan;26(1):1–9. PubMed PMID: 17209691.

Holman AJ, Myers RR. A randomized, double-blind, placebo-controlled trial of pramipexole, a dopamine agonist, in patients with fibromyalgia receiving concomitant medications. Arthritis Rheum. 2005 Aug;52(8):2495–505. PubMed PMID: 16052595.

Holton KF, Taren DL, Thomson CA, Bennett RM, Jones KD. The effect of dietary glutamate on fibromyalgia and irritable bowel symptoms. Clin Exp Rheumatol. 2012 Nov–Dec;30(6 Suppl 74):10–17. PubMed PMID: 22766026.

Hsieh LF, Hong CZ, Chern SH, Chen CC. Efficacy and side effects of diclofenac patch in treatment of patients with myofascial pain syndrome of the upper trapezius. J Pain Symptom Manage. 2010 Jan;39(1):116–25. PubMed PMID: 19822404.

Kararizou E, Anagnostou E, Triantafyllou NI. Dramatic improvement of fibromyalgia symptoms after treatment with topiramate for coexisting migraine. J Clin Psychopharmacol. 2013 Oct;33(5):721–23. PubMed PMID: 23948791.

Kleinböhl D, Görtelmeyer R, Bender HJ, Hölzl R. Amantadine sulfate reduces experimental sensitization and pain in chronic back pain patients. Anesth Analg. 2006 Mar;102(3):840–47. PubMed PMID: 16492838.

Lee YC, Nassikas NJ, Clauw DJ. The role of the central nervous system in the generation and maintenance of chronic pain in rheumatoid arthritis, osteoarthritis and fibromyalgia. Arthritis Res Ther. 2011 Apr 28;13(2):211. PubMed PMID: 21542893.

Light KC, Bragdon EE, Grewen KM, Brownley KA, Girdler SS, Maixner W. Adrenergic dysregulation and pain with and without acute beta-blockade in women with fibromyalgia and temporomandibular disorder. J Pain. 2009 May;10(5):542–52. PubMed PMID: 19411061.

Lynch ME, Clark AJ, Sawynok J, Sullivan MJ. Topical amitriptyline and ketamine in neuropathic pain syndromes: an open-label study. J Pain. 2005 Oct;6(10):644–49. PubMed PMID: 16202956.

McCleane G. Does intravenous lidocaine reduce fibromyalgia pain? A randomized, double-blind, placebo controlled crossover study. The Pain Clinic. 2000;12(3):181–85.

Murphy SL, Phillips K, Williams DA, Clauw DJ. The role of the central nervous system in osteoarthritis pain and implications for rehabilitation. Curr Rheumatol Rep. 2012 Dec;14(6):576–82. PubMed PMID: 22879060.

Oaklander AL, Herzog ZD, Downs HM, Klein MM. Objective evidence that small-fiber polyneuropathy underlies some illnesses currently labeled as fibromyalgia. Pain. 2013 Nov; 154(11):2310–16. PubMed PMID: 23748113.

Olivan-Blázquez B, Herrera-Mercadal P, Puebla-Guedea M, Pérez-Yus MC, Andrés E, Fayed N, López-Del-Hoyo Y, Magallon R, Roca M, Garcia-Campayo J. Efficacy of memantine in the treatment of fibromyalgia: a double-blind, randomised, controlled trial with 6-month follow-up. Pain. 2014 Dec; 155(12):2517–25. PubMed PMID: 25218600.

Prescrire Int. Fibromyalgia: poorly understood; treatments are disappointing. 2009 Aug;18(102):169–73. PubMed PMID: 19746561.

Radley DC, Finkelstein SN, Stafford RS. Off-label prescribing among office-based physicians. Arch Intern Med. 2006 May 8; 166(9):1021–26. PubMed PMID: 16682577.

Raphael JH, Southall JL, Kitas GD. Adverse effects of intravenous lignocaine [lidocaine] therapy in fibromyalgia syndrome. Rheumatology (Oxford). 2003 Jan;42(1):185–86. PubMed PMID: 12509636.

Recla JM, Sarantopoulos CD. Combined use of pregabalin and memantine in fibromyalgia syndrome treatment: a novel analgesic and neuroprotective strategy? Med Hypotheses. 2009 Aug;73(2):177–83. PubMed PMID: 19362430.

Schafranski MD, Malucelli T, Machado F, Takeshi H, Kaiber F, Schmidt C, Harth F. Intravenous lidocaine for fibromyalgia syndrome: an open trial. Clin Rheumatol. 2009 Jul;28(7):853–55. PMID: 19263182.

Smith JD, Terpening CM, Schmidt SO, Gums JG. Relief of fibromyalgia symptoms following discontinuation of dietary excitotoxins. Ann Pharmacother. 2001 Jun;35(6):702–6. PubMed PMID: 11408989.

Sörensen J, Bengtsson A, Bäckman E, Henriksson KG, Bengtsson M. Pain analysis in patients with fibromyalgia. Effects of intravenous morphine, lidocaine, and ketamine. Scand J Rheumatol. 1995;24(6):360–65. PubMed PMID: 8610220.

Stoschitzky K, Sakotnik A, Lercher P, Zweiker R, Maier R, Liebmann P, Lindner W. Influence of beta-blockers on melatonin release. Eur J Clin Pharmacol. 1999 Apr;55(2):111–15. PubMed PMID: 10335905.

Taylor AG, Anderson JG, Riedel SL, Lewis JE, Bourguignon C. A randomized, controlled, double-blind pilot study of the effects of cranial electrical stimulation on activity in brain pain processing regions in individuals with fibromyalgia. Explore (NY). 2013 Jan–Feb;9(1):32–40. PubMed PMID: 23294818.

Tegeder I, Muth-Selbach U, Lötsch J, Rüsing G, Oelkers R, Brune K, Meller S, Kelm GR, Sörgel F, Geisslinger G. Application of microdialysis for the determination of muscle and subcutaneous tissue concentrations after oral and topical ibuprofen administration. Clin Pharmacol Ther. 1999 Apr;65(4):357–68. PubMed PMID: 10223771.

Tremont-Lukats IW, Challapalli V, McNicol ED, Lau J, Carr DB. Systemic administration of local anesthetics to relieve neuropathic pain: a systematic review and meta-analysis. Anesth Analg. 2005 Dec;101(6):1738–49. PubMed PMID: 16301253.

Üçeyler N, Zeller D, Kahn AK, Kewenig S, Kittel-Schneider S, Schmid A, Casanova-Molla J, Reiners K, Sommer C. Small fibre pathology in patients with fibromyalgia syndrome. Brain. 2013 Jun;136(Pt 6):1857–67. PubMed PMID: 23474848.

Üçeyler N, Sommer C, Walitt B, Häuser W. Anticonvulsants for fibromyalgia. Cochrane Database Syst Rev. 2013 Oct 16;10: CD010782. PubMed PMID: 24129853.

Uzaraga I, Gerbis B, Holwerda E, Gillis D, Wai E. Topical amitriptyline, ketamine, and lidocaine in neuropathic pain caused by radiation skin reaction: a pilot study. Support Care Cancer. 2012 Jul;20(7):1515–24. PubMed PMID: 21847539.

Watkins LR, Hutchinson MR, Ledeboer A, Wieseler-Frank J, Milligan ED, Maier SF. Glia as the "bad guys": implications for improving clinical pain control and the clinical utility of opioids. Brain Behav Immun. 2007 Feb;21(2):131–46. PubMed PMID: 17175134.

Wood PB, Kablinger AS, Caldito GS. Open trial of pindolol in the treatment of fibromyalgia. Ann Pharmacother. 2005 Nov;39(11):1812–16. PubMed PMID: 16219901.

Younger J, Noor N, McCue R, Mackey S. Low-dose naltrexone for the treatment of fibromyalgia: findings of a small, randomized, double-blind, placebo-controlled, counterbalanced, crossover trial assessing daily pain levels. Arthritis Rheum. 2013 Feb;65(2):529–38. PubMed PMID: 23359310.

Younger J, Parkitny L, McLain D. The use of low-dose naltrexone (LDN) as a novel anti-inflammatory treatment for chronic pain. Clin Rheumatol. 2014 Apr;33(4):451–59. PubMed PMID: 24526250.

Yunus MB, Masi AT, Aldag JC. Short term effects of ibuprofen in primary fibromyalgia syndrome: a double blind, placebo controlled trial. J Rheumatol. 1989 Apr;16(4):527–32. PubMed PMID: 2664173.

Ziegler D, Nowak H, Kempler P, Vargha P, Low PA. Treatment of symptomatic diabetic polyneuropathy with the antioxidant alpha-lipoic acid: a meta-analysis. Diabet Med. 2004 Feb; 21(2):114–21. PubMed PMID: 14984445.

Ziegler D, Ametov A, Barinov A, Dyck PJ, Gurieva I, Low PA, Munzel U, Yakhno N, Raz I, Novosadova M, Maus J, Samigullin R. Oral treatment with alpha-lipoic acid improves symptomatic diabetic polyneuropathy: the SYDNEY 2 trial. Diabetes Care. 2006 Nov;29(11):2365–70. PubMed PMID: 17065669.

Chapter 20. Reduce: Opiates for Pain Relief

Baron MJ, McDonald PW. Significant pain reduction in chronic pain patients after detoxification from high-dose opioids. J Opioid Manag. 2006 Sep–Oct;2(5):277–82.

Bennett RM, Kamin M, Karim R, Rosenthal N. Tramadol and acetaminophen combination tablets in the treatment of fibromyalgia pain: a double-blind, randomized, placebo-controlled study. Am J Med. 2003 May;114(7):537–45. PubMed PMID: 12753877.

Benyamin R, Trescot AM, Datta S, Buenaventura R, Adlaka R, Sehgal N, Glaser SE, Vallejo R. Opioid complications and side effects. Pain Physician. 2008 Mar;11(2 Suppl):S105–20.

Berger A, Sadosky A, Dukes EM, Edelsberg J, Zlateva G, Oster G. Patterns of healthcare utilization and cost in patients with newly diagnosed fibromyalgia. Am J Manag Care. 2010 May;16(5 Suppl):S126–37. PubMed PMID: 20586521.

Fitzcharles MA, Ste-Marie PA, Gamsa A, Ware MA, Shir Y. Opioid use, misuse, and abuse in patients labeled as fibromyalgia. Am J Med. 2011 Oct;124(10):955–60. PubMed PMID: 21962316.

Fitzcharles MA, Faregh N, Ste-Marie PA, Shir Y. Opioid use in fibromyalgia is associated with negative health related measures in a prospective cohort study. Pain Res Treat. 2013; 2013:898493. PubMed PMID: 23577251.

Kemple, KL, Smith G, Wong-Ngan J. Opioid therapy in fibromyalgia: a four year prospective evaluation of therapy selection, efficacy, and predictions of outcome. Arthritis Rheum. 2003; 48:S88.

Koppert W, Ihmsen H, Körber N, Wehrfritz A, Sittl R, Schmelz M, Schüttler J. Different profiles of buprenorphine-induced analgesia and antihyperalgesia in a human pain model. Pain. 2005 Nov;118(1–2):15–22. PubMed PMID:16154698.

Lee M, Silverman SM, Hansen H, Patel VB, Manchikanti L. A comprehensive review of opioid-induced hyperalgesia. Pain

Physician. 2011 Mar–Apr;14(2):145–61. PubMed PMID: 21412369.

Russell IJ, Kamin M, Bennett RM, Schnitzer TJ, Green JA, Katz WA. Efficacy of tramadol in treatment of pain in fibromyalgia. J Clin Rheumatol. 2000 Oct;6(5):250–57. PubMed PMID: 19078481.

Salpeter SR, Buckley JS, Bruera E. The use of very-low-dose methadone for palliative pain control and the prevention of opioid hyperalgesia. J Palliat Med. 2013 Jun;16(6):616–22. PubMed PMID: 23556990.

Shaw IR, Lavigne G, Mayer P, Choinière M. Acute intravenous administration of morphine perturbs sleep architecture in healthy pain-free young adults: a preliminary study. Sleep. 2005 Jun;28(6):677–82. PubMed PMID: 16477954.

Sörensen J, Bengtsson A, Bäckman E, Henriksson KG, Bengtsson M. Pain analysis in patients with fibromyalgia. Effects of intravenous morphine, lidocaine, and ketamine. Scand J Rheumatol. 1995;24(6):360–65. PubMed PMID: 8610220.

Chapter 21. Reduce: Medical Marijuana for Pain Relief

Blake DR, Robson P, Ho M, Jubb RW, McCabe CS. Preliminary assessment of the efficacy, tolerability and safety of a cannabis-based medicine (Sativex) in the treatment of pain caused by rheumatoid arthritis. Rheumatology (Oxford). 2006 Jan;45(1): 50–52. PubMed PMID: 16282192.

Burstein SH, Zurier RB. Cannabinoids, endocannabinoids, and related analogs in inflammation. AAPS J. 2009 Mar;11(1): 109–19. PubMed PMID: 19199042.

Costa B, Trovato AE, Comelli F, Giagnoni G, Colleoni M. The non-psychoactive cannabis constituent cannabidiol is an orally effective therapeutic agent in rat chronic inflammatory and neuropathic pain. Eur J Pharmacol. 2007 Feb 5;556(1–3):75–83. PubMed PMID: 17157290.

Dietrich A, McDaniel WF. Endocannabinoids and exercise. Br J Sports Med. 2004 Oct;38(5):536–41. Review. PubMed PMID: 15388533.

Fiz J, Durán M, Capellà D, Carbonell J, Farré M. Cannabis use in patients with fibromyalgia: effect on symptoms relief and health-related quality of life. PLoS One. 2011 Apr 21;6(4):e18440. PubMed PMID: 21533029.

Garcia-Gonzalez E, Selvi E, Balistreri E, Lorenzini S, Maggio R, Natale MR, Capecchi PL, Lazzerini PE, Bardelli M, Laghi-Pasini F, Galeazzi M. Cannabinoids inhibit fibrogenesis in diffuse systemic sclerosis fibroblasts. Rheumatology (Oxford). 2009 Sep;48(9):1050–56. PubMed PMID: 19589890.

Mack A, Joy J. Marijuana as medicine?: the science beyond the controversy. Washington, DC: National Academies Press, 2000.

McPartland JM. Expression of the endocannabinoid system in fibroblasts and myofascial tissues. J Bodyw Mov Ther. 2008 Apr;12(2):169–82. PubMed PMID: 19083670.

McPartland JM, Giuffrida A, King J, Skinner E, Scotter J, Musty RE. Cannabimimetic effects of osteopathic manipulative treatment. J Am Osteopath Assoc. 2005 Jun;105(6):283–91. PubMed PMID: 16118355.

Manzanares J, Julian M, Carrascosa A. Role of the cannabinoid system in pain control and therapeutic implications for the management of acute and chronic pain episodes. Curr Neuropharmacol. 2006 Jul;4(3):239–57. PubMed PMID: 18615144.

Mao J, Price DD, Lu J, Keniston L, Mayer DJ. Two distinctive antinociceptive systems in rats with pathological pain. Neurosci Lett. 2000 Feb 11;280(1):13–16. PubMed PMID: 10696800.

Nackley AG, Zvonok AM, Makriyannis A, Hohmann AG. Activation of cannabinoid CB2 receptors suppresses C-fiber responses and windup in spinal wide dynamic range neurons in the absence and presence of inflammation. J Neurophysiol. 2004 Dec;92(6):3562–74. PubMed PMID: 15317842.

Rog DJ, Nurmikko TJ, Friede T, Young CA. Randomized, controlled trial of cannabis-based medicine in central pain in multiple sclerosis. Neurology. 2005 Sep 27;65(6):812–19. PubMed PMID: 16186518.

Schley M, Legler A, Skopp G, Schmelz M, Konrad C, Rukwied R. Delta-9-THC based monotherapy in fibromyalgia patients on experimentally induced pain, axon reflex flare, and pain relief. Curr Med Res Opin. 2006 Jul;22(7):1269–76. PubMed PMID: 16834825.

Skrabek RQ, Galimova L, Ethans K, Perry D. Nabilone for the treatment of pain in fibromyalgia. J Pain. 2008 Feb;9(2):164–73. PubMed PMID:17974490.

Sparling PB, Giuffrida A, Piomelli D, Rosskopf L, Dietrich A. Exercise activates the endocannabinoid system. Neuroreport. 2003 Dec 2;14(17):2209–11. PubMed PMID: 14625449.

Ste-Marie PA, Fitzcharles MA, Gamsa A, Ware MA, Shir Y. Association of herbal cannabis use with negative psychosocial parameters in patients with fibromyalgia. Arthritis Care Res (Hoboken). 2012 Aug;64(8):1202–8. PubMed PMID: 22730275.

Sumariwalla PF, Gallily R, Tchilibon S, Fride E, Mechoulam R, Feldmann M. A novel synthetic, nonpsychoactive cannabinoid acid (HU-320) with antiinflammatory properties in murine collagen-induced arthritis. Arthritis Rheum. 2004 Mar;50(3): 985–98. PubMed PMID: 15022343.

Wade DT, Robson P, House H, Makela P, Aram J. A preliminary controlled study to determine whether whole-plant cannabis extracts can improve intractable neurogenic symptoms. Clin Rehabil. 2003 Feb;17(1):21–29. PubMed PMID: 12617376.

Walker JM, Hohmann AG, Martin WJ, Strangman NM, Huang SM, Tsou K. The neurobiology of cannabinoid analgesia. Life Sci. 1999;65(6–7):665–73. PubMed PMID: 10462067.

Wallace M, Schulteis G, Atkinson JH, Wolfson T, Lazzaretto D, Bentley H, Gouaux B, Abramson I. Dose-dependent effects of smoked cannabis on capsaicin-induced pain and hyperalgesia in healthy volunteers. Anesthesiology. 2007 Nov;107(5):785–96. PubMed PMID: 18073554.

Walter L, Franklin A, Witting A, Wade C, Xie Y, Kunos G, Mackie K, Stella N. Nonpsychotropic cannabinoid receptors regulate microglial cell migration. J Neurosci. 2003 Feb 15;23(4):1398–405. PubMed PMID: 12598628.

Ware MA, Fitzcharles MA, Joseph L, Shir Y. The effects of nabilone on sleep in fibromyalgia: results of a randomized controlled trial. Anesth Analg. 2010 Feb 1;110(2):604–10. PubMed PMID: 20007734.

Ware MA, Wang T, Shapiro S, Robinson A, Ducruet T, Huynh T, Gamsa A, Bennett GJ, Collet JP. Smoked cannabis for chronic neuropathic pain: a randomized controlled trial. CMAJ. 2010 Oct 5;182(14):E694–701. PubMed PMID: 20805210.

Chapter 22. Reduce: Pain from Other Sources

Ametov AS, Barinov A, Dyck PJ, Hermann R, Kozlova N, Litchy WJ, Low PA, Nehrdich D, Novosadova M, O'Brien PC, Reljanovic M, Samigullin R, Schuette K, Strokov I, Tritschler HJ, Wessel K, Yakhno N, Ziegler D; SYDNEY Trial Study Group. The sensory symptoms of diabetic polyneuropathy are improved with alpha-lipoic acid: the SYDNEY trial. Diabetes Care. 2003 Mar;26(3):770–76. PubMed PMID: 12610036.

Amris K, Jespersen A, Bliddal H. Self-reported somatosensory symptoms of neuropathic pain in fibromyalgia and chronic widespread pain correlate with tender point count and pressure-pain thresholds. Pain. 2010 Dec;151(3):664–69. PubMed PMID: 20832941.

Baraf HS, Gold MS, Clark MB, Altman RD. Safety and efficacy of topical diclofenac sodium 1% gel in knee osteoarthritis: a randomized controlled trial. Phys Sportsmed. 2010 Jun;38(2): 19–28. PubMed PMID: 20631460.

Barthel HR, Haselwood D, Longley S 3rd, Gold MS, Altman RD. Randomized controlled trial of diclofenac sodium gel in knee osteoarthritis. Semin Arthritis Rheum. 2009 Dec;39(3): 203–12. PubMed PMID: 19932833.

Belcaro G, Cesarone MR, Dugall M, Pellegrini L, Ledda A, Grossi MG, Togni S, Appendino G. Efficacy and safety of Meriva®, a curcumin-phosphatidylcholine complex, during extended administration in osteoarthritis patients. Altern Med Rev. 2010 Dec;15(4):337–44. PubMed PMID: 21194249.

FitzGerald MP, Payne CK, Lukacz ES, Yang CC, Peters KM, Chai TC, Nickel JC, Hanno PM, Kreder KJ, Burks DA, Mayer R, Kotarinos R, Fortman C, Allen TM, Fraser L, Mason-Cover M, Furey C, Odabachian L, Sanfield A, Chu J, Huestis K, Tata

GE, Dugan N, Sheth H, Bewyer K, Anaeme A, Newton K, Featherstone W, Halle-Podell R, Cen L, Landis JR, Propert KJ, Foster HE Jr, Kusek JW, Nyberg LM; Interstitial Cystitis Collaborative Research Network. Randomized multicenter clinical trial of myofascial physical therapy in women with interstitial cystitis/painful bladder syndrome and pelvic floor tenderness. J Urol. 2012 Jun;187(6):2113–18. PubMed PMID: 22503015.

Giannoccaro MP, Donadio V, Incensi A, Avoni P, Liguori R. Small nerve fiber involvement in patients referred for fibromyalgia. Muscle Nerve. 2014 May;49(5):757–59. PubMed PMID: 24469976.

Jacobs AM, Cheng D. Management of diabetic small-fiber neuropathy with combination L-methylfolate, methylcobalamin, and pyridoxal 5'-phosphate. Rev Neurol Dis. 2011;8(1–2):39–47. PubMed PMID: 21769070.

Lee JD, Park HJ, Chae Y, Lim S. An Overview of Bee Venom Acupuncture in the Treatment of Arthritis. Evid Based Complement Alternat Med. 2005 Mar;2(1):79–84. PubMed PMID: 15841281.

Lee MS, Pittler MH, Shin BC, Kong JC, Ernst E. Bee venom acupuncture for musculoskeletal pain: a review. J Pain. 2008 Apr;9(4):289–97. PubMed PMID: 18226968.

Manheimer E, Cheng K, Linde K, Lao L, Yoo J, Wieland S, van der Windt DA, Berman BM, Bouter LM. Acupuncture for peripheral joint osteoarthritis. Cochrane Database Syst Rev. 2010 Jan 20;(1):CD001977. PubMed PMID: 20091527.

Oaklander AL, Herzog ZD, Downs HM, Klein MM. Objective evidence that small-fiber polyneuropathy underlies some illnesses currently labeled as fibromyalgia. Pain. 2013 Nov; 154(11):2310–16. PubMed PMID: 23748113.

Parsons CL. The role of the urinary epithelium in the pathogenesis of interstitial cystitis/prostatitis/urethritis. Urology. 2007 Apr;69(4 Suppl):9–16. PubMed PMID: 17462486.

Pertovaara A. The noradrenergic pain regulation system: a potential target for pain therapy. Eur J Pharmacol. 2013 Sep 15;716(1–3):2–7. PubMed PMID: 23500194.

Roth SH, Shainhouse JZ. Efficacy and safety of a topical diclofenac solution (pennsaid) in the treatment of primary osteoarthritis of the knee: a randomized, double-blind, vehicle-controlled clinical trial. Arch Intern Med. 2004 Oct 11;164(18):2017–23. PubMed PMID: 15477437.

van Ophoven A, Pokupic S, Heinecke A, Hertle L. A prospective, randomized, placebo controlled, double-blind study of amitriptyline for the treatment of interstitial cystitis. J Urol. 2004 Aug;172(2):533–36. PubMed PMID: 15247722.

Walker MJ Jr, Morris LM, Cheng D. Improvement of cutaneous sensitivity in diabetic peripheral neuropathy with combination L-methylfolate, methylcobalamin, and pyridoxal 5'-phosphate. Rev Neurol Dis. 2010;7(4):132–39. PubMed PMID: 21206429.

Weiss JM. Pelvic floor myofascial trigger points: manual therapy for interstitial cystitis and the urgency-frequency syndrome. J Urol. 2001 Dec;166(6):2226–31. PubMed PMID: 11696740.

Ziegler D, Nowak H, Kempler P, Vargha P, Low PA. Treatment of symptomatic diabetic polyneuropathy with the antioxidant alpha-lipoic acid: a meta-analysis. Diabet Med. 2004 Feb;21(2): 114–21. PubMed PMID: 14984445.

Ziegler D, Ametov A, Barinov A, Dyck PJ, Gurieva I, Low PA, Munzel U, Yakhno N, Raz I, Novosadova M, Maus J, Samigullin R. Oral treatment with alpha-lipoic acid improves symptomatic diabetic polyneuropathy: the SYDNEY 2 trial. Diabetes Care. 2006 Nov;29(11):2365–70. PubMed PMID: 17065669.

Chapter 23. Reduce: Chronic Fatigue Syndrome

Arora R, Chawla R, Marwah R, Arora P, Sharma RK, Kaushik V, Goel R, Kaur A, Silambarasan M, Tripathi RP, Bhardwaj JR. Potential of complementary and alternative medicine in preventive management of novel H1N1 flu (swine flu) pandemic: thwarting potential disasters in the bud. Evid Based Complement Alternat Med. 2011;2011:586506. PubMed PMID: 20976081.

Bennett AL, Mayes DM, Fagioli LR, Guerriero R, Komaroff AL. Somatomedin C (insulin-like growth factor I) levels in patients with chronic fatigue syndrome. J Psychiatr Res. 1997 Jan–Feb;31(1):91–66. PubMed PMID: 9201651.

Bradley AS, Ford B, Bansal AS. Altered functional B cell subset populations in patients with chronic fatigue syndrome compared to healthy controls. Clin Exp Immunol. 2013 Apr; 172(1):73–80. PubMed PMID: 23480187.

Broderick G, Fuite J, Kreitz A, Vernon SD, Klimas N, Fletcher MA. A formal analysis of cytokine networks in chronic fatigue syndrome. Brain Behav Immun. 2010 Oct;24(7):1209–17. PubMed PMID: 20447453.

Brook MG, Bannister BA, Weir WR. Interferon-alpha therapy for patients with chronic fatigue syndrome. J Infect Dis. 1993 Sep;168(3):791–92. PubMed PMID: 8354926.

Chia JK. The role of enterovirus in chronic fatigue syndrome. J Clin Pathol. 2005 Nov;58(11):1126–32. PubMed PMID: 16254097.

Evengard B, Nilsson CG, Lindh G, Lindquist L, Eneroth P, Fredrikson S, Terenius L, Henriksson KG. Chronic fatigue syndrome differs from fibromyalgia. No evidence for elevated substance P levels in cerebrospinal fluid of patients with chronic fatigue syndrome. Pain. 1998 Nov;78(2):153–55. PubMed PMID: 9839828.

Fluge Ø, Bruland O, Risa K, Storstein A, Kristoffersen EK, Sapkota D, Næss H, Dahl O, Nyland H, Mella O. Benefit from B-lymphocyte depletion using the anti-CD20 antibody rituximab in chronic fatigue syndrome. A double-blind and placebo-controlled study. PLoS One. 2011;6(10):e26358. PubMed PMID: 22039471.

Fukuda K, Straus SE, Hickie I, Sharpe MC, Dobbins JG, Komaroff A. The chronic fatigue syndrome: a comprehensive approach to its definition and study. International Chronic Fatigue Syndrome Study Group. Ann Intern Med. 1994 Dec 15;121(12):953–59. PubMed PMID: 7978722.

Garcia MN, Hause AM, Walker CM, Orange JS, Hasbun R, Murray KO. Evaluation of prolonged fatigue post–West Nile virus infection and association of fatigue with elevated antiviral and proinflammatory cytokines. Viral Immunol. 2014 Sep; 27(7):327–33. PubMed PMID: 25062274.

IOM (Institute of Medicine). Beyond myalgic encephalomyelitis/ chronic fatigue syndrome: redefining an illness. Report guide for clinicians. 2015. http://iom.nationalacademies.org /~/media/Files/Report%20Files/2015/MECFS/MECFS cliniciansguide.pdf.

Hornig M, Montoya JG, Klimas NG, Levine S, Felsenstein D, Bateman L, Peterson DL, Gottschalk CG, Schultz AF, Che X, Eddy ML, Komaroff AL, Lipkin WI. Distinct plasma immune signatures in ME/CFS are present early in the course of illness. Sci Adv. 2015 Feb;1(1). PubMed PMID: 26079000.

Hornung B, Amtmann E, Sauer G. Lauric acid inhibits the maturation of vesicular stomatitis virus. J Gen Virol. 1994 Feb;75(Pt 2):353–61. PubMed PMID: 8113756.

Kendall SA, Schaadt ML, Graff LB, Wittrup I, Malmskov H, Krogsgaard K, Bartels EM, Bliddal H, Danneskiold-Samsøe B. No effect of antiviral (valacyclovir) treatment in fibromyalgia: a double blind, randomized study. J Rheumatol. 2004 Apr;31(4): 783–84. PubMed PMID: 15088307.

Knox K, Carrigan D, Simmons G, Teque F, Zhou Y, Hackett J Jr, Qiu X, Luk KC, Schochetman G, Knox A, Kogelnik AM, Levy JA. No evidence of murine-like gammaretroviruses in CFS patients previously identified as XMRV-infected. Science. 2011 Jul 1;333(6038):94–97. PubMed PMID: 21628393.

Kogelnik AM, Loomis K, Hoegh-Petersen M, Rosso F, Hischier C, Montoya JG. Use of valganciclovir in patients with elevated antibody titers against Human Herpesvirus-6 (HHV-6) and Epstein-Barr Virus (EBV) who were experiencing central nervous system dysfunction including long-standing fatigue. J Clin Virol. 2006 Dec;37 Suppl 1:S33–38. PubMed PMID: 17276366.

Lerner AM, Zervos M, Chang CH, Beqaj S, Goldstein J, O'Neill W, Dworkin H, Fitzgerald T, Deeter RG. A small, randomized, placebo-controlled trial of the use of antiviral therapy for patients with chronic fatigue syndrome. Clin Infect Dis. 2001 Jun 1;32(11):1657–58. PubMed PMID: 11340544.

Lerner AM, Beqaj SH, Deeter RG, Fitzgerald JT. Valacyclovir treatment in Epstein-Barr virus subset chronic fatigue syndrome: thirty-six months follow-up. In Vivo. 2007 Sep–Oct; 21(5):707–13. PubMed PMID: 18019402.

Loebel M, Strohschein K, Giannini C, Koelsch U, Bauer S, Doebis C, Thomas S, Unterwalder N, von Baehr V, Reinke P, Knops

M, Hanitsch LG, Meisel C, Volk HD, Scheibenbogen C. Deficient EBV-specific B- and T-cell response in patients with chronic fatigue syndrome. PLoS One. 2014 Jan 15;9(1):e85387. PubMed PMID: 24454857.

Lombardi VC, Ruscetti FW, Das Gupta J, Pfost MA, Hagen KS, Peterson DL, Ruscetti SK, Bagni RK, Petrow-Sadowski C, Gold B, Dean M, Silverman RH, Mikovits JA. Detection of an infectious retrovirus, XMRV, in blood cells of patients with chronic fatigue syndrome. Science. 2009 Oct 23;326(5952):585–89. PubMed PMID: 19815723.

Montoya JG, Kogelnik AM, Bhangoo M, Lunn MR, Flamand L, Merrihew LE, Watt T, Kubo JT, Paik J, Desai M. Randomized clinical trial to evaluate the efficacy and safety of valganciclovir in a subset of patients with chronic fatigue syndrome. J Med Virol. 2013 Dec;85(12):2101–9. PubMed PMID: 23959519.

Moorkens G, Wynants H, Abs R. Effect of growth hormone treatment in patients with chronic fatigue syndrome: a preliminary study. Growth Horm IGF Res. 1998 Apr;8 Suppl B:131–33. PubMed PMID: 10990148.

Rosenbaum ME, Vojdani A, Susser M, Watson CM. Improved immune activation markers in chronic fatigue and immune dysfunction syndrome (CFIDS) patients treated with thymic protein A. J Nutr Environ Med. 2001;11(4):241–47.

Satterfield BC, Garcia RA, Jia H, Tang S, Zheng H, Switzer WM. Serologic and PCR testing of persons with chronic fatigue syndrome in the United States shows no association with xenotropic or polytropic murine leukemia virus–related viruses. Retrovirology. 2011 Feb 22;8:12. PubMedPMID: 21342521.

Scharf MB, Baumann M, Berkowitz DV. The effects of sodium oxybate on clinical symptoms and sleep patterns in patients with fibromyalgia. J Rheumatol. 2003 May;30(5):1070–74. PubMed PMID: 1273490.

See DM, Tilles JG. Alpha-interferon treatment of patients with chronic fatigue syndrome. Immunol Invest. 1996 Jan–Mar; 25(1–2):153–64. PubMed PMID: 8675231.

Straus SE. The chronic mononucleosis syndrome. J Infect Dis. 1988 Mar;157(3):405–12. PubMed PMID: 2830340.

Strayer DR, Carter WA, Brodsky I, Cheney P, Peterson D, Salvato P, Thompson C, Loveless M, Shapiro DE, Elsasser W, et al. A controlled clinical trial with a specifically configured RNA drug, poly(I).poly(C12U), in chronic fatigue syndrome. Clin Infect Dis. 1994 Jan;18 Suppl 1:S88–95. PubMed PMID: 8148460.

Strayer DR, Carter WA, Stouch BC, Stevens SR, Bateman L, Cimoch PJ, Lapp CW, Peterson DL; Chronic Fatigue Syndrome AMP-516 Study Group, Mitchell WM. A double-blind, placebo-controlled, randomized, clinical trial of the TLR-3 agonist rintatolimod in severe cases of chronic fatigue syndrome. PLoS One. 2012;7(3):e31334. PMID: 22431963.

Watt T, Oberfoell S, Balise R, Lunn MR, Kar AK, Merrihew L, Bhangoo MS, Montoya JG. Response to valganciclovir in chronic fatigue syndrome patients with human herpesvirus 6 and Epstein-Barr virus IgG antibody titers. J Med Virol. 2012 Dec;84(12):1967–74. PubMed PMID: 23080504.

Wysenbeek AJ, Shapira Y, Leibovici L. Primary fibromyalgia and the chronic fatigue syndrome. Rheumatol Int. 1991; 10(6):227–29. PubMed PMID: 2041979.

INDEX

Page numbers of illustrations appear in italics.

ABOUT THE AUTHOR

GINEVRA LIPTAN, M.D., is a graduate of Tufts University School of Medicine and board-certified in internal medicine. Formerly an associate professor at Oregon Health & Science University, she is now medical director of the Frida Center for Fibromyalgia, a fibromyalgia specialty clinic (www .fridacenter.com). The clinic is named for Frida Kahlo, the Mexican artist, who endured years of chronic pain and is thought to have been a fibromyalgia sufferer.

Dr. Liptan is the medical advisor to the Fibromyalgia Information Foundation and is on the board of the Mastering Pain Institute. She received a Gerlinger Foundation research award to study myofascial release for fibromyalgia, with results published in the *Journal of Bodywork and Movement Therapies*. She has also published articles in peer-reviewed medical journals about fibromyalgia exercise and self-management strategies. She is married to her high school sweetheart, Jamie, a myofascial release therapist, with a daughter named Samantha. They live in multigenerational and multispecies housing in the wonderfully weird city of Portland, Oregon.

ABOUT THE TYPE

This book was set in Minion, a 1990 Adobe Originals typeface by Robert Slimbach (b. 1956). Minion is inspired by classical, old-style typefaces of the late Renaissance, a period of elegant, beautiful, and highly readable type designs. Created primarily for text setting, Minion combines the aesthetic and functional qualities that make text type highly readable with the versatility of digital technology.